Nutritional Biochemistry

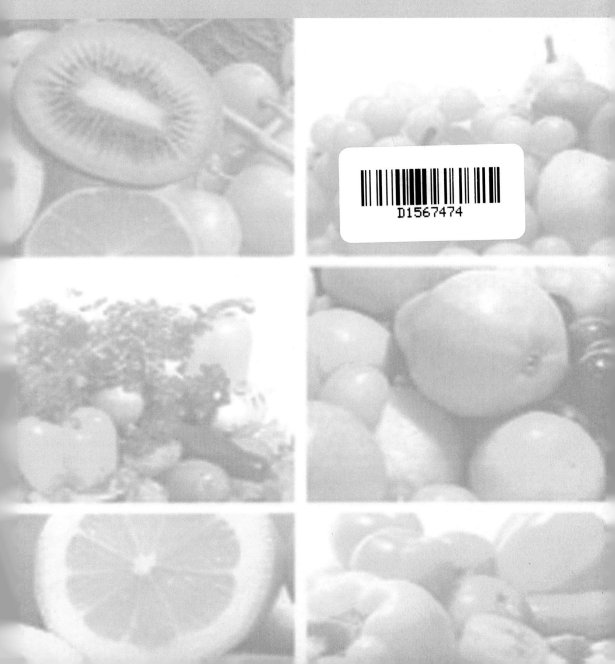

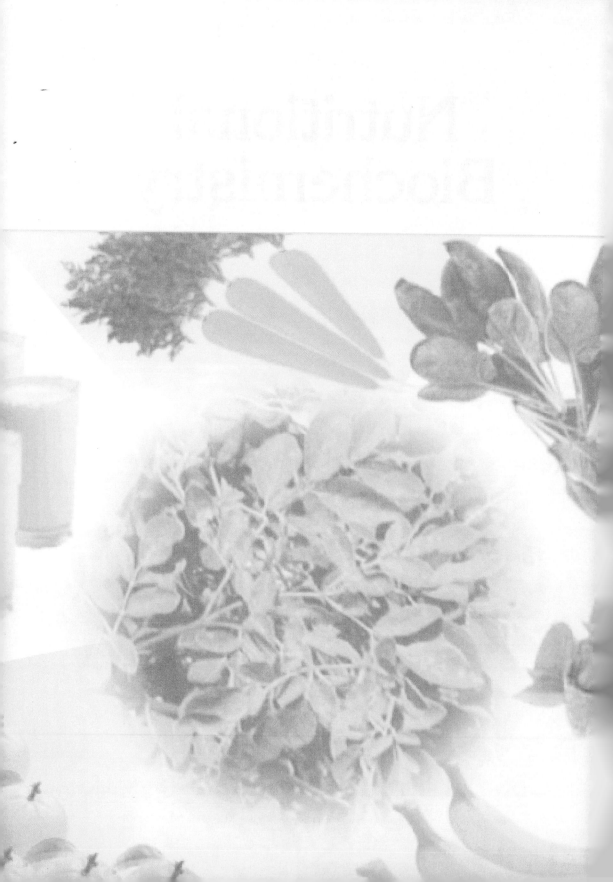

Nutritional Biochemistry

DC Sharma

MSc, PhD (Bio), PhD (Med)

Ex-Professor and Head
Department of Biochemistry
Government Medical Colleges
Jaipur, Kangra, Bikaner and Agroha
and
SGT Dental College, Budhera, Gurgaon

Devanshi Sharma

MSc (Clinical nutrition)

Clinical Nutritionist
Fortis Hospital, Gurgaon

CBS

CBS Publishers & Distributors Pvt Ltd

New Delhi • Bengaluru • Chennai • Kochi • Kolkata • Mumbai
Hyderabad • Nagpur • Patna • Pune • Vijayawada

Disclaimer

Science and technology are constantly changing felds. New research and experience broaden the scope of information and knowledge. The authors have tried their best in giving information available to them while preparing the material for this book. Although, all efforts have been made to ensure optimum accuracy of the material, yet it is quite possible some errors might have been left uncorrected. The publisher, the printer and the authors will not be held responsible for any inadvertent errors or inaccuracies.

Nutritional Biochemistry

ISBN: 978-81-239-2527-1

First Edition: 2015
Reprint: 2017

Published by Satish Kumar Jain and produced by Varun Jain for
CBS Publishers & Distributors Pvt Ltd
4819/XI Prahlad Street, 24 Ansari Road, Daryaganj, New Delhi 110 002, India.
Ph: 23289259, 23266861, 23266867 Website: www.cbspd.com
Fax: 011-23243014 e-mail: delhi@cbspd.com; cbspubs@airtelmail.in.
Corporate Office: 204 FIE, Industrial Area, Patparganj, Delhi 110 092
Ph: 4934 4934 Fax: 4934 4935 e-mail: publishing@cbspd.com; publicity@cbspd.com

Branches

- **Bengaluru:** Seema House 2975, 17th Cross, K.R. Road, Banasankari 2nd Stage, Bengaluru 560 070, Karnataka
  Ph: +91-80-26771678/79 Fax: +91-80-26771680 e-mail: bangalore@cbspd.com
- **Chennai:** 7, Subbaraya Street, Shenoy Nagar, Chennai 600 030, Tamil Nadu
  Ph: +91-44-26680620, 26681266 Fax: +91-44-42032115 e-mail: chennai@cbspd.com
- **Kochi:** Ashana House, No. 39/1904, AM Thomas Road, Valanjambalam, Ernakulam 682 018, Kochi, Kerala
  Ph: +91-484-4059061-62-64-65 Fax: +91-484-4059065 e-mail: kochi@cbspd.com
- **Kolkata:** 6/B, Ground Floor, Rameswar Shaw Road, Kolkata-700 014, West Bengal
  Ph: +91-33-22891126, 22891127, 22891128 e-mail: kolkata@cbspd.com
- **Mumbai:** 83-C, Dr E Moses Road, Worli, Mumbai-400018, Maharashtra
  Ph: +91-22-24902340/41 Fax: +91-22-24902342 e-mail: mumbai@cbspd.com

Representatives

- **Hyderabad** 0-9885175004 • **Nagpur** 0-9021734563 • **Patna** 0-9334159340
- **Pune** 0-9623451994 • **Vijayawada** 0-9000660880

Printed at: India Binding House, Noida, UP

Preface

Biochemistry is the core subject of all medical and biological sciences. Since it is the study of chemistry of living things, there has to be a variety of subject books depending upon the course of study, for example, plant biochemistry, animal biochemistry, human biochemistry and biochemistry of micro-organisms—bacteria and viruses, etc. Naturally, the contents of each of these branches will be different.

A textbook has to be "tailor made" according to the standard of the students and requirements of a particular course of study. A book good for a particular course may not necessarily be good for another course. Unfortunately, there is practically no book on biochemistry for the students of nutrition and they are required to study textbooks meant for medical or dental students. Although the biochemistry is same, each book is different from the other in treatment, extent and emphasis as per the course. A book meant for medical students is more detailed and clinically oriented while the nutrition students require knowledge on basic biochemistry with emphasis on food sources of all the nutrients (carbohydrates, proteins, fats, lipids, vitamins and minerals). Keeping this in view, the first author has endeavoured to write this book for BSc (nutrition) and BSc (home science) courses, while he has to his credit several books for medical, dental and nursing students. In this task, he was ably assisted by the second author, who herself obtained BSc and MSc degrees in nutrition and is working as a clinical nutritionist for more than two years in one of the leading hospitals in Gurgaon.

The authors are thankful to Dr Jai Ram Rawtani, Associate Professor, Medical College, Jodhpur, for reviewing some of the chapters of this book.

It is earnestly hoped that this book will truly serve its purpose for which it was written.

DC Sharma
Devanshi Sharma

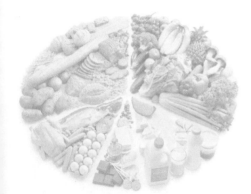

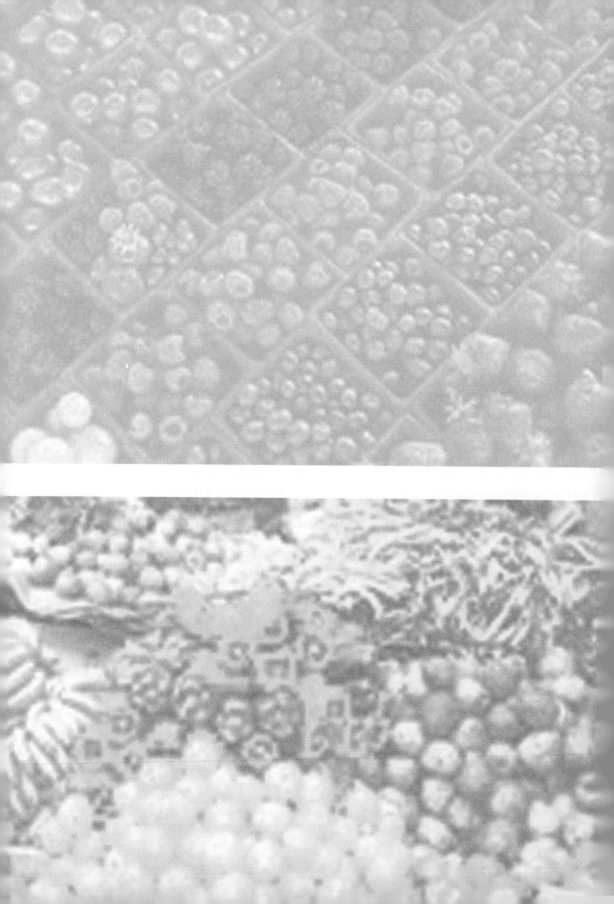

Contents

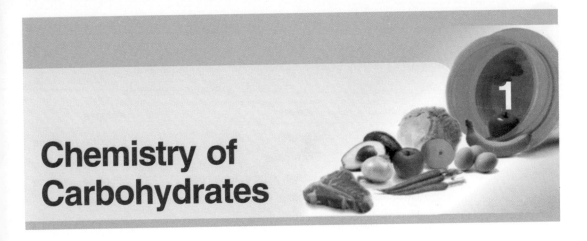

Chemistry of Carbohydrates

INTRODUCTION

Carbohydrates are sugar and starch-like substances which ordinarily contain carbon, hydrogen and oxygen. Their modern definition is based on the understanding of their structure, so carbohydrates are defined as compounds which contain aldehyde or ketone group and a number of alcoholic groups or if it is capable of producing such a substance on hydrolysis. Generally, these are defined as polyhydroxy aldehydes or ketones or their derivatives.

–CHO		–CO
Aldehyde group		Keto group
–CH$_2$OH	–CHOH	–CHO
Primary	Secondary	Tertiary
	Alcoholic groups	

CLASSIFICATION

From early times, two distinct types of carbohydrates are recognised mainly on the basis of their physical properties. These are sugars (like cane sugar, glucose and fructose) and starches (rice starch, potato starch).

Sugars: These are generally simple low molecular weight substances, soluble in water, sweet in taste, are mainly crystalline, have reducing nature.

Starches: These are complex high molecular weight substances, insoluble in water or give colloidal solution, are neither sweet in taste nor reducing in nature. Some of them give varying color with iodine.

However, modern classification of carbohydrates as well as proteins and lipids, is based on the understanding of products of their hydrolysis. In this way, carbohydrates are classified into three categories on the basis of number of simple sugar units produced on hydrolysis.

1. **Monosaccharides:** 'Mono' means one and 'saccharides' means sugar units, so those carbohydrates which are made up of only one sugar unit and cannot be further hydrolyzed into simpler form, are termed as monosaccharides. Their general formula is $C_nH_{2n}O_n$, where 'n' is the number of carbon atoms. They are further subdivided into trioses (3), tetroses (4), pentoses (5), hexoses (6) and heptoses (7), on the basis of number of carbon atoms present. Alternatively, they have been sub-classified into aldoses or ketoses on the basis of functional group, which is aldehyde in an aldose and ketone group in a ketose. Glucose and fructose are their respective examples.

   Different types of monosaccharides are found in food (Table 1.1).

2. **Disaccharides:** 'Di' means two so disaccharides are those carbohydrates which contain two simple sugar units which are liberated on hydrolysis. Sucrose, lactose and maltose are well known examples of disaccharides. They

Table 1.1: Different types of monosaccharides found in food

Monosaccharides		Specific examples	
No. of carbon atoms	Called as	Aldoses	Ketoses
Three	Trioses	Glycerol	Dihydroxyacetone
Four	Tetroses	Erythroses	Erythrulose
Five	Pentoses	Ribose, xylose, arabinose	Ribulose, xylulose
Six	Hexoses	Glucose, galactose, mannose	Fructose
Seven	Heptoses	Glucoheptose	Sedoheptulose

are represented by general formula $C_n(H_2O)_{n-1}$.

3. **Polysaccharides:** 'Poly' means many, so polysaccharides are made up of many simple sugar units. Generally this number is very high, so polysaccharides are those carbohydrates which on complete hydrolysis, produce a large number of simple sugar units. They are called hexosan or pentosan depending on whether it is a polymer of a hexose or a pentose. Similarly, they are known as glucosan or fructosan depending on whether glucose or fructose is present as a repeating unit.

Occurrence: A large number of carbohydrates occur in nature. We shall study only those which occur in the human body or the food (Table 1.2). Some common carbohydrates of food in the form of sugar and starches are shown in Fig. 1.1.

MONOSACCHARIDES

All carbohydrates are made up of one or more monosaccharides. Therefore, the structure of monosaccharides will be discussed first taking glucose as an example which is by far the most important carbohydrate. The molecule of glucose is basically an aldohexose. Different forms of its structure have been suggested by different workers.

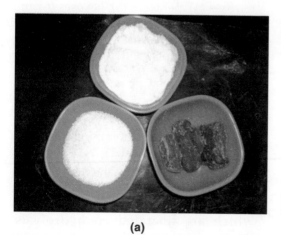

(a)

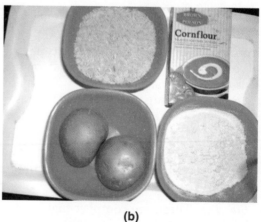

(b)

Fig. 1.1: (a) Food sources of carbohydrates (sugars) and **(b)** food sources of carbohydrates (starches)

Table 1.2: Commonly occurring carbohydrates and their sources	
Carbohydrates	*Sources*
Monosaccharides	
Glucose	Blood sugar, fruits, honey, grapes; in combined form in starches and dextrins, and sucrose, lactose, maltose.
Fructose	Fruits, honey; in combined form in inulin and sucrose.
Galactose	In lactose and brain lipids in combination.
Pentose	Fruit juices, nucleic acids.
Disaccharides	
Lactose (milk sugar)	Milk
Sucrose (cane sugar)	Cane juice, table sugar, sweets, beet sugar and pineapple.
Maltose (malt sugar)	Malt; formed during hydrolysis of starch and dextrin and germination of cereals.
Polysaccharides	
Starch	Cereals, tubers, roots and pulses; acts as reserve carbohydrate in plants. Rice and potatoes are very rich sources.
Dextrin	Cereals, tubers, roots and pulses; formed by partial hydrolysis of starch in the gut.
Glycogen	Liver, muscle; acts as reserve carbohydrate in animals.
Cellulose	Plants; acts as structural constituent of plants (plant fibers).

a. Straight chain structure

D-Glucose   L-Glucose   D-Fructose   D-Galactose   D-Mannose

b. Ring structure

α-D-Glucopyranose   Open chain glucose   β-D-Glucopyranose

c. Ring structure with pyranose and furanose form

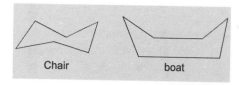

d. Ring pyranose form structure in 'chair' and 'boat' configuration

For the sake of simplicity, we shall use straight chain structure (a) or straight chain with ring formation (b).

Isomerism: It can be seen from structures (a) that glucose contains four asymmetric carbon atoms (carbon no. 2, 3, 4 and 5). The presence of an asymmetric carbon atom gives rise to the possibility of stereo-isomerism. The number of possible isomers is calculated by formula 2^n, where 'n' is the number of asymmetric carbon atoms. Since glucose has four asymmetric carbon atoms, it exists in $2^4 = 16$, forms. Half (8) are mirror images of other half (8). The orientation of H and OH groups on penultimate carbon determines the family to which sugar belongs. If –OH group is in right side, the sugar belongs to D-family; if –OH is on left side, it belongs to L-family. Note that all natural sugars are of D-family.

- **Aldose-ketose isomerism:** The monosaccharide having aldehyde group is called aldose, while having ketone group is called ketose. Glucose and fructose both have same formula $C_6H_{12}O_6$ but glucose is a aldohexose (aldehyde bearing hexose) and fructose is a ketohexose (ketone bearing hexose), so they are isomers of one another (Fig. 1.2).

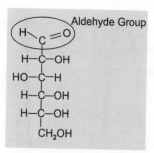

Fig. 1.2: Aldose-ketose isomerism

- **Stereoisomerism:** Stereoisomerism occurs when the same compounds due to different spatial arrangement of the groups attached to its asymmetric carbon atom or chiral carbon atom [a carbon atom to which four different groups or atoms attached (marked in Fig. 1.3 with an*)] exists in more than one form. Thus, monosaccharides have two different forms namely 'D-sugar' and 'L-sugar', depending on their relation to the direction of the –OH group on the last but one carbon atom.

The D-sugars have –OH group attached on the right side of that carbon atom and L-sugars have –OH group attached on the left side of that carbon atom. The simplest three carbon naturally occurring glycerides (Fig. 1.3) lack a plane of symmetry and exist as a pair of *Enantiomers* (stereoisomerism that are mirror image of one another) D and L forms. The majority of the mono-saccharides occurring in mammalian tissues are of D-configuration.

Another type of stereoisomerism known as *Epimerism* occurs with respect to a single asymmetric carbon atom of a mono-saccharide possessing more than one asymmetric carbon atoms. In Fig. 1.4, there

$$\xleftarrow{\text{Left}} \quad \overset{1}{C}HO \atop HO—\overset{2}{C^*}—H \atop \overset{3}{C}H_2OH \qquad \overset{1}{C}HO \atop H—\overset{2}{C^*}—OH \atop \overset{3}{C}H_2OH \xrightarrow{\text{Right}}$$

Fig. 1.3: Structural isomerism of glyceraldehydes

Note: * chiral carbon atom

are six carbon (hexose) sugars. Four carbon atoms (C-2, C-3, C-4 and C-5) are chiral atoms. These are structural isomers, i.e. they have the same molecular formulae of $C_6H_{12}O_6$, but different structural formula, and consequently they differ in physical and chemical properties. These isomers are formed by interchange of the –OH and –H on carbon atoms 2, 4 of glucose. Glucose and galactose differ in the configuration of a single carbon atom (C-4) while glucose and mannose differ at carbon atom no. 2, as indicated in Fig. 1.4. Compounds that differ in this manner are called *epimers*.

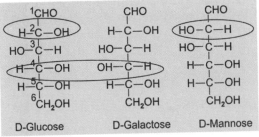

D-Glucose   D-Galactose   D-Mannose

Fig. 1.4: Epimers: Glucose, galactose and mannose

Optical Activity

The presence of asymmetric carbon atom in a compound also confers optical activity, i.e. such substances when in solution are able to rotate the plane of plane polarized light. The optical rotation may be clockwise (dextro) or anticlockwise (levo) and the substance is

called dextrorotatory or levorotatory, respectively (Fig. 1.5). The optical rotation can be measured in degrees in an instrument called 'polarimeter' and expressed by putting prefix d or (+) for dextrorotation and l or (–) for levorotation. Glucose is dextrorotatory while fructose is levorotatory.

Properties

The properties of a molecule are manifestation of its structure. We shall discuss important properties of monosaccharides taking glucose as an example.

Physical Properties

Glucose and other sugars are soluble in water, generally sweet in taste and are mainly crystalline. They exhibit isomerism and optical activity.

Chemical Properties

Glucose show several chemical reactions which are either due to carbonyl group or hydroxylic groups or the whole molecule. We shall discuss only important properties.

1. *Reducing action:* One of the most notable property of glucose and other monosaccharides, is their reducing action, that is, they are able to reduce several ions in hot alkaline medium. The most notable is reduction of cupric ions to cuprous ions as in Benedict's test. The glucose is

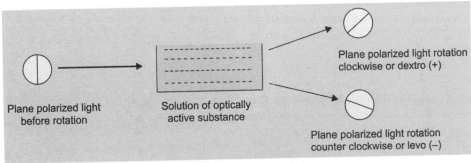

Plane polarized light before rotation

Solution of optically active substance

Plane polarized light rotation clockwise or dextro (+)

Plane polarized light rotation counter clockwise or levo (–)

Fig. 1.5: Optical rotation

simultaneously oxidized to gluconic acid in which aldehyde group is converted into carboxylic group. It is possible to oxidize terminal alcoholic group of glucose protecting aldehyde group. The resulting compound is glucuronic acid, which still possesses the reducing property, on account of free aldehyde group. When both the terminal groups are oxidized, saccharic acid is formed. Galactose on the other hand, gives mucic acid.

2. *Osazone formation:* Osazones are yellow or orange crystalline derivatives of reducing sugars with phenyl hydrazine. They have characteristic crystal structure and definite melting points. The crystal structure can be seen under microscope and is used for identification and characterization of the sugars. However, glucose, fructose and mannose form same osazone but different from that of galactose.

$$D\text{-(+) glucose} \longrightarrow \text{(fructose)}$$
$$D\text{-osazone} \longleftarrow D\text{-(+) mannose}$$

3. *Esterification:* The alcoholic groups of glucose react with acids like phosphoric acid which are physiologically very important compounds, e.g. glucose-6-phosphate.

$$\text{D-glucose + phosphoric acid} \longrightarrow$$
$$\text{D-glucose-6-phosphate} + H_2O$$

4. *Glycoside formation:* Glycosides are formed when a carbohydrate combines with a non-carbohydrate. The non-carbohydrate is called aglycone. It may be methyl alcohol, glycerol, a sterol or phenol. A simple example is formation of methyl glycoside, by boiling a solution of glucose with methyl alcohol in presence of HCl as a catalyst. Many drugs and spices contain glycosides. Some of them are digitalis, phlorhizin and saponin. All of them contain a steroid as an aglycone.

5. *Amination:* The replacement of hydroxylic group of glucose or other mono-saccharide by amino group gives amino sugars. Various amino sugars are found in body as a part of mucopolysaccharides. For example, glucosamine is a part of hyaluronic acid, galactosamine of chondroitin and mannosamine of mucoprotein. Several antibiotics (e.g. erythromycin, carbomycin) also contain amino sugar, which moiety is responsible for their antibiotic activity.

DISACCHARIDES

When two monosaccharides combine together, a water molecule is eliminated and the two units join together by a characteristic bond called glycosidic bond (–o–). Depending on the nature of monosaccharides present, different disaccharides are formed as highlighted in Table 1.3.

Table 1.3: Constituents of disaccharides

Disaccharides	Monosaccharides present
Maltose	Glucose (two molecules)
Lactose	Glucose, galactose
Sucrose	Glucose, fructose

The important disaccharides are maltose (glucose-o-glucose by α-1, 4 glycosidic linkage) (Fig. 1.6a), lactose (glucose-o-galactose by α, β-1, 4 glycosidic linkage) (Fig. 1.6b) and sucrose (glucose-o-fructose by α, β-1, 2 glycosidic linkage) (Fig. 1.6c).

Maltose

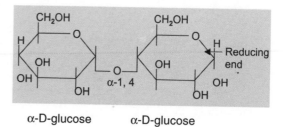

α-D-glucose   α-D-glucose

Fig. 1.6a: Maltose

Lactose

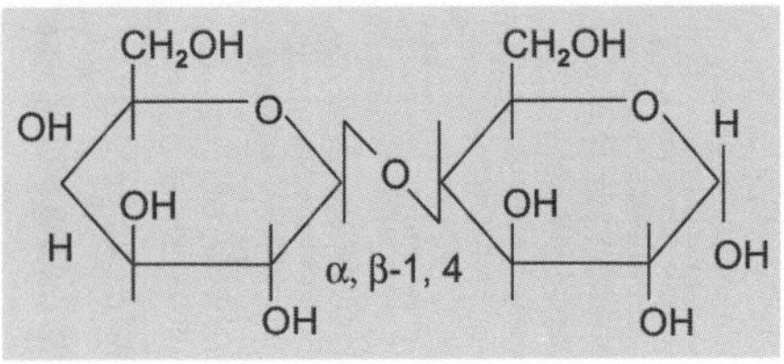

CH₂OH   CH₂OH

OH   O   O   H

OH   OH

H   α, β-1, 4   OH

OH   OH

β-D-galactose   α-D-glucose

Fig. 1.6b: Lactose

Sucrose

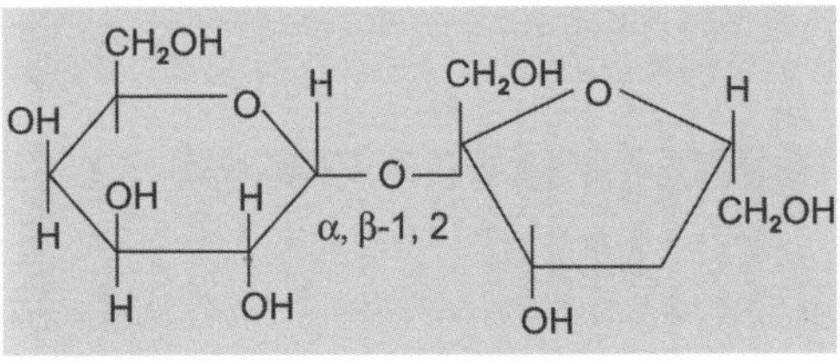

CH₂OH   H   CH₂OH   O   H

OH   O

OH   H   O   CH₂OH

H   α, β-1, 2

H   OH   OH

α-D-glucose   β-D-fructose

Fig. 1.6c: Sucrose

Maltose is found in malt, also formed in germinating cereals and in gut by digestion of starch and dextrin. Lactose is found in milk, formed by lactating mammary glands and sometimes passed in urine by pregnant or lactating females. Sucrose is most widely consumed as sugar. It mainly occurs in cane juice. It is non-reducing as none of the carbonyl group of either monosaccharide is free. For the same reason, it does not form an osazone.

POLYSACCHARIDES

Polysaccharides are polymers of many monosaccharide units. Polysaccharides are produced when many monosaccharide units are joined together by glycosidic linkage. Important ones are cellulose, starch, dextrin and glycogen. They are all polymers of glucose, hence, are also called glucosan. Inulin is a polymer of fructose, so it is known as fructosan.

Chemically, polysaccharides are of two types:

a. *Homopolysaccharides or homoglycans* which possess only one type of monosaccharides, such as starch, cellulose, etc.

b. *Heteropolysaccharides or heteroglycans* which are formed by more than one type of monosaccharides, such as hyaluronic acid and heparin. Table 1.4 lists the commonly occurring polysaccharides of different types.

Homopolysaccharides

Cellulose

It is the chief constituent of plant cell wall and most common and abundant of the D-glucose polymers, but does not occur in human tissues. It is made up of a large number of glucose units. It is homopolymers of glucose like starch. Cellulose form cell wall of vegetables, fruits and cereals. Cattle can digest and utilize cellulose but the humans cannot.

The adjacent glucose units in cellulose molecules are joined by a glycosidic linkage between first carbons of one unit to fourth carbon of next glucose unit. The glucose units of cellulose are β-glucose because –OH group on carbon no. 1 is on the right side as opposed to –OH group on the left side present in other polysaccharides (Fig. 1.7). All glucose units are joined in straight chain-like structure forming fibers. Cotton and paper are nearly pure cellulose. Cellulose is insoluble in water due to intra- and inter-chain hydrogen bonds. It is not

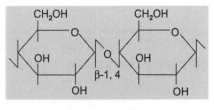

CH₂OH   CH₂OH

O   O

OH   O   OH

β-1, 4

OH   OH

Glucose   Glucose

Fig. 1.7: Repeating units of cellulose

Table 1.4: Constituents of common polysaccharides

Polysaccharides	Examples	Monosaccharides presents
Homopolysaccharides	Starch	Glucose
	Cellulose	Glucose
	Glycogen	Glucose
	Dextrins	Glucose
	Inulin	Fructose
	Pectins	Methyl D-galactouronate
Heteropolysaccharides	Hyaluronic acid	Glucoronic acid, N-acetylglucosamine
	Chondroitin sulphate	Glucoronic acid, 2-N-acetylaminogalactose
	Heparin	Glucosamine, glucuronic acid

degraded by amylases of salivary or pancreatic juice because of β-orientation of –OH group on carbon no. 1 of glucose moiety. Hence, dietary cellulose is passed as such in the stool as its "bulk". Constipated person can be helped by the cellulose. The presence of cellulose in diet stimulates peristalsis which ensures normal bowel movements and easy defecation. A soluble derivative of cellulose (carboxymethylcellulose) has been prepared and is used for slimming.

A liberal intake of foods containing cellulose, such as wheat bran, leafy vegetables and fruits is helpful. Wheat flour from which bran has been removed contains little cellulose and provides less bulk in the intestine. Brown bread made from whole wheat flour is more helpful in cases of constipation than white bread prepared from flour devoid of bran. Isabgol is cellulose with a capacity to absorb over 25 times its weight of water. It is extensively used for treating constipation.

Starch

Starch is the most important food source amongst carbohydrates and is principally found in potatoes, rice, cereals and pulses. It is actually a mixture of two polysaccharides—amylose and amylopectin; the proportion of these two in natural starch varies with the food source.

a. Amylose

i. The proportion of amylose in natural starch ranges from 10–20%.

ii. It is made up of 200–2000 glucose units.

iii. The glucose units are joined together by α-1, 4 linkage as in maltose.

iv. It is soluble in boiling water.

b. Amylopectin

i. Its proportion in normal starch varies from 80–90%.

ii. It contains 250–5000 glucose units.

iii. The glucose units are joined by α-1, 4 linkage up to about 24 units and then branching occurs by α-1, 6 linkage.

iv. It is insoluble in boiling water.

Cooking facilitate digestion of starch. Boiling causes swelling of the starch granules and rupture of the cell walls, thus allowing better digestion. *Farina* is dried potato starch. *Sago* is prepared from the trunk of the sago palm (Metroxylon sago). Sago is essential starch. Yams greater yam (Dioscorea alata) and lesser yams (Descuenta) are big and small tubers of climbing tropical plants and are rich in starch.

The enzyme amylase, present in salivary and pancreatic juice, converts starch into maltose which is broken into glucose which gets absorbed. Starch present in some unripe fruits is converted into glucose which gives a sweet taste.

Dextrins

These are also polymers of D-glucose held by α (1–4) glycosidic linkage. Dextrins are, in fact, formed due to partial hydrolysis of starch by enzymes, such as salivary amylase, dilute mineral acids or heat. Dextrins form sticky solution in water and are frequently used as adhesives, e.g. on postage stamps. They may have feeble reducing properties and when hydrolyzed, yield maltose and finally glucose.

Dextrins are also formed in gut or in cooking. They give reddish violet color with iodine. Various dextrins have been described depending upon the complexity of molecule. Erythrodextrins or limit dextrins give red color with iodine. Further hydrolysis yield achrodextrins which give no color with iodine. Finally only reducing sugars remain.

Glycogen

It is the storage polysaccharide found in the muscles and liver of animals and humans. Glycogen resembles amylopectin, but it is highly branched (Fig. 1.8). The branches occur after 8–12 glucose units by α-1, 6-linkage. Thus, its structure very much resembles that of a tree. It has about 25000 glucose units; the molecular weight is around 5 millions. It forms colloidal solution which gives red color with iodine. Glycogen acts as reserve carbohydrate in animals that means it serves to store energy in the form of glucose residues.

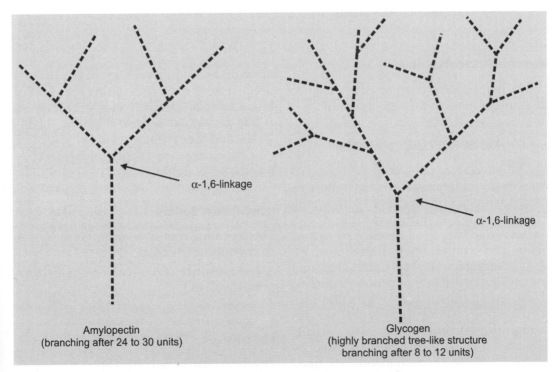

α-1,6-linkage

α-1,6-linkage

Amylopectin
(branching after 24 to 30 units)

Glycogen
(highly branched tree-like structure branching after 8 to 12 units)

Fig. 1.8: Branching in amylopectin and glycogen

Inulin: Inulin is a plant polysaccharide made up of fructose and is soluble in warm water. It does not give any color with iodine. It has sweet taste and present in many vegetables and fruits including onion, leeks, banana, asparagus, etc. (Fig. 1.9).

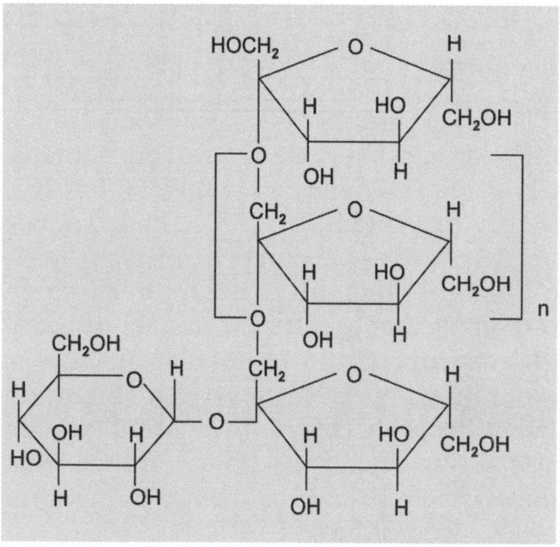

Fig. 1.9: Inulin (n = approx. 35)

Heteropolysaccharides

Unlike homopolysaccharides, these contain dissimilar sugars in the repeating unit.

MUCOPOLYSACCHARIDES

Unlike polysaccharides, mucopolysaccharides or glycosaminoglycans are built from more than one type of carbohydrate unit. Thus, they are complex carbohydrates characterized by the presence of uronic acids and aminated, sulfated and N-acetylated sugars. They are found in ground (or packing) substance of connective tissue (bone, elastin and collagen) where they play a structural role. Mucopolysaccharides containing uronic acids are acidic. Mucopolysaccharides when attached by covalent bond to a protein (core) are termed as 'proteoglycans'.

Due to the presence of large number of –OH groups and negative charges on the mucopolysaccharide molecules, they have property of holding large quantities of water and occupying space, which make them suitable for cushioning or lubricating other structures.

Blood group substances are mucopolysaccharides which confer blood typing to RBCs in blood group determination. Some important mucopolysaccharides are described below:

Hyaluronic Acid

Hyaluronate or hyaluronic acid contains 400–4000 units of repeating unit. The molecular weight is around 1.5×10^5 to 1.5×10^6. It coils and forms gel, so it acts as a lubricant in synovial fluid present in bone joints. The repeating unit of hyaluronic acid is:

[Glucuronic acid-N-acetylglucosamine]

It is replaced in adult life by less elastic dermatan sulfate.

Heparin

Heparin is a powerful anticoagulant. It is derived from mast cells, lining the walls of blood vessels, especially in liver and lungs. It has molecular weight around 15,000–20,000 and the repeating unit is:

[Glucuronic acid-2-sulfate-glucosamine-6-sulfate-2-N-sulfate]

Chondroitin Sulfate

The repeating unit of chondroitin sulfate A or chondroitin-4-sulfate is:

[Glucuronic acid-N-acetylgalactosamine-4-sulfate]

DIETARY FIBER

The diet contains not only above mentioned carbohydrates but also several compounds

Table 1.5: Food sources of dietary fiber

Cellulose	Hemicellulose	Pectin
Whole wheat flour	Cereals	Apples
Cabbage	Whole grains	Citrus fruits
Peas	Guar gum	Vegetables
Beans	Oatmeal	Strawberries
Apples	Wheat	
Root vegetables	Beans	
Legumes		

of this group which neither gives energy in the body nor serves as structural constituents of body structure. They are, in fact, part of structure of plant tissues, and are called fiber components. They are however, useful in human nutrition for maintaining intestinal motility and clear bowel movement. Additionally, they help reduce blood sugar and cholesterol. We have given food sources of various fiber components in Table 1.5.

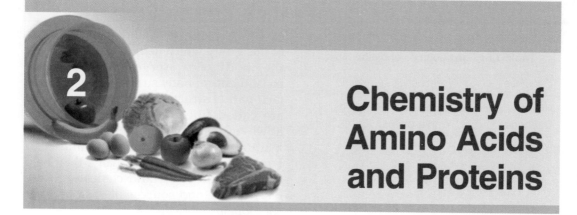

Chemistry of Amino Acids and Proteins

2

INTRODUCTION

The building blocks of proteins are amino acids. In order to understand proteins, it is important to know amino acids. All amino acids essentially contain carbon, hydrogen, oxygen and nitrogen and some contain sulphur.

AMINO ACIDS

An amino acid is a compound in which carboxylic as well as amino group is attached to the same carbon atom. Their general formula is written as $R.CHNH_2.COOH$. The different amino acids differ with respect to R-group.

Classification

The 20 naturally occurring amino acids are classified on the basis of R-group as given below:

i. *Amino acid with aliphatic R-group:* Glycine, alanine, valine, leucine, isoleucine, methionine, proline and cysteine are of this category.

ii. *Amino acid with aromatic R-group:* Phenylalanine, tyrosine and tryptophan are of this type.

iii. *Polar amino acid having charged R-group:* Arginine, lysine, histidine, aspartic acid and glutamic acid belong to this class.

iv. *Polar amino acid with neutral or uncharged R-group:* Serine, threonine, asparagine

and glutamine are included in this group.

Some Important Amino Acids

Glycine: This is the simplest amino acid. Glycine is necessary for the formation of the bile acid, glycocholic acid and glutathione. It can be utilized to form ribose, glucose, fatty acids, aspartic acid, purine, pyrimidine and porphyrin structure of heme for the formation of hemoglobin.

Tyrosine: The thyroid gland utilizes tyrosine and iodine for the formation of monoiodotyrosine, diiodotyrosine and the hormone thyroxine. The hormone adrenalin and the pigment melanin are also synthesized from tyrosine.

Lysine: It is necessary for growth. A diet consisting mainly of rice and wheat is deficient in lysine and has to be supplemented by milk and soyabean, both of which are rich in lysine.

Tryptophan: It is partially converted to nicotinamide in the body. About 60 mg of tryptophan is equivalent to 1 mg nicotinamide. Thus, tryptophan helps to prevent pallegra.

Methionine: It contains a methyl group and sulphur. The methyl group helps to form choline which is called lipotropic factor because it removes fat from the liver. Methionine is abundant in milk protein, casein. The methionine content of cereals and pulses is low. Sesame seeds, used for producing sesame oil, are rich in methionine.

Cystin and cysteine: Cystin and cysteine are other sulphur containing amino acids. Cysteine is converted in cystine by oxidation and condensation of two molecules of the former. Insulin is rich in cystin.

Phenylalanine: It is a precursor of the amino acid tyrosine and thus aids in the formation of the hormone adrenalin and thyroxine and the pigment melanin. The mental retardation in childhood occurs as an inborn error of metabolism phenylketonuria due to deficiency of enzyme—phenylhydroxylase.

Histidine: It is essential for the growth and repair of human tissues. Histidine can be converted into histamine which, when released in the skin, produces urticaria rash.

Leucine: It depresses blood sugar in most individuals. It inhibits the liver output of glucose and stimulates pancreatic insulin secretion. Some people, who are more sensitive to leucine, develop low blood sugar and even convulsion with dietary leucine. In such cases, protein restriction and high carbohydrate diet help. A diet high in leucine (maize, jowar) tends to produce pellagra.

Arginine: This amino acid, essential to children but not to adults, is a constituent of many proteins, including albumin. In addition, it is made in the body during the synthesis of urea in the liver from ammonia and carbon dioxide.

Alanine: This is the main glucogenic amino acid that is converted by the liver into glucose (gluconeogenesis). This mechanism maintains the blood glucose level in fasting state. The non-essential amino acids are degraded in muscles to form alanine. Insulin inhibits alanine formation and fasting accelerates its formation in the muscles.

PROPERTIES OF AMINO ACIDS

Physical Properties

The properties of a compound depend on its structure. Since amino acids are ionic compounds, they are generally soluble in polar solvents (water), have high melting points ($> 200°C$) and are crystalline. Except glycine, all amino acids are optically active due to presence of asymmetric carbon atom.

Solubility: Amino acids are readily soluble in water, slightly soluble in ethanol and insoluble in ether. Tyrosine is soluble in hot water but sparingly soluble in cold water. Cysteine is soluble with difficulty in only hot water. Proline and hydroxyl proline are soluble in alcohol and ether.

Amino acids are generally soluble in acids and bases and form salts. Tyrosine is moderately soluble in acids and bases. Cysteine is soluble in strong mineral acids (HCl) but slightly soluble in acetic acid and dilute ammonia.

Taste: Amino acids are sweet, tasteless or bitter. Histidine is sweet, leucine is tasteless, whereas isoleucine and arginine are bitter in taste.

Sodium salt of glutamic acid (monosodium glutamate, MSG, also known as Ajinomoto) is valuable as a flavoring agent for certain food (for meat and meat products and sauces) because it imparts and enhances the flavor.

Optical Properties

Stereochemistry of Amino Acids

All amino acids (except glycine) rotate the plane of plane polarized light because of the presence of asymmetric carbon at C-2. Both L (amino group on left side) and D (amino group on right side) enantiomers are

L-amino acid   D-amino acid

possible for the amino acids. However, all the amino acids in the diet and in the body occur as L form.

Chemical Properties

A few important chemical properties are described here.

i. *Peptide bond formation:* As the amino acids have oppositely charged groups, two amino acids can combine to form a compound called di-peptide having a peptide (CO.NH) bond. This reaction can be repeated several times giving rise to tripeptide, tetrapeptide and polypeptides, etc. and serves to form complex proteins.

$$NH_3^+CH_2COO^- + NH_3^+CH_2COO^- \longrightarrow H_2O +$$
$$NH_3^+CH_2CONH.CH_2COO^-$$
$$\text{Di-peptide}$$

ii. *Ionization:* Another important property of amino acids is ionization. Amino acids possess one free amino and one free carboxylic group. These groups are ionizable, hence, extent of ionization will vary depending on pH of medium. In neutral solution, these groups are fully ionized and exist as NH_3^+ and COO^-. But the net charge on the molecule is zero. In acidic medium, the amino acid exists as a cation (NH_3^+) because acids being proton donors donate proton to COO^- ion and nullify its charge. Hence, the net charge on the molecule is (+1). In alkaline medium, the alkalis being proton acceptor, accept a proton from NH_3^+ group. The net charge on the molecule becomes (−1), hence, amino acid acts as an anion.

Some amino acids have more than two ionizable groups (glutamic acid, arginine), hence, the net charge on the molecule will be more and will vary accordingly to the pH of the medium. The pH at which the net charge is zero or minimum is known as isoelectric pH.

iii. *Decarboxylation:* On heating with barium hydroxide, the carboxylic group of amino acid is removed as CO_2 and amino acid form amine.

$$R-CH-COOH \longrightarrow R-CH_2-NH_2 + CO_2$$
$$NH_2$$

Amino acid   Amine

Decarboxylation reaction

The decarboxylation reaction is very important in the body as it serves to form many physiologically active amine compounds (e.g. serotonin, histamine and dopamine) some of which act as neurotransmitters. The decarboxylation reaction also occurs in intestine. After a heavy protein meal, amino acids still present in the gut are acted upon by bacterial enzyme (decarboxylase) to yield respective amine, many of which are toxic. They are called ptomaines. These are responsible for sick feeling observed after protein indigestion.

iv. *Nitrous acid reaction:* When treated with nitrous acid, amino acids yield nitrogen gas which can be trapped and volume measured. This is one of the methods of estimating amino acid nitrogen.

$$H_3N^+-\underset{\underset{H}{|}}{\overset{\overset{R}{|}}{C}}-COOH \underset{}{\overset{H^+}{\rightleftharpoons}} H_3N^+-\underset{\underset{H}{|}}{\overset{\overset{R}{|}}{C}}-COO^- \underset{}{\overset{H^+}{\rightleftharpoons}} H_2N-\underset{\underset{H}{|}}{\overset{\overset{R}{|}}{C}}-COO^-$$

In acidic soln.   In neutral soln.   In alkaline soln.
net charge (+1)   net charge (0)   net charge (−1)
cation   dipolar ion   anion

Ionization

v. *Formol titration:* Formaldehyde when added to a solution of amino acid masks its amino group, thus making it possible to titrate carboxylic group with an alkali.

vi. *Ninhydrin reaction:* Many amino acids react with ninhydrin (triketohydrindene hydrate) to give blue or purple colored compounds. This reaction is very useful in detection of minute quantities of amino acids by chromatographic technique.

vii. *Sanger's reaction:* Sanger discovered that the compound 1-fluoro-2, 4-dinitrobenzene (DNB), reacts with free amino group of amino acid or protein to form intense yellow DNP-amino acid. This reaction has helped in determining the sequence of amino acids in many proteins and polypeptide chains. Because of its importance, the reaction is known as, Sanger's reaction and the reagent as Sanger's reagent. Using this reaction, Sanger determined the complete structure of insulin hormone for which he was awarded Nobel Prize.

POLYPEPTIDES

Polypeptides are chains of amino acids held together by peptide bonds. Two amino acids link to form a dipeptide, three a tripeptide and so on. When the amino acids are up to 10, then peptide is called oligopeptide. Beyond that, it is polypeptide. Each peptide begins with an amino terminal and ends with a free carboxyl terminal.

Among the various existing peptides, some are especially important from the physiological point of view. These are:

Glutathione: It is a tripeptide made up of glutamic acid, cysteine and glycine. The compound is involved in oxidation-reduction reaction.

Oxytocin and vasopressin: These peptide hormones of the pituitary gland consist of 8 amino acids. These aid in the ejection of milk and water re-absorption in the kidney, respectively, besides other functions.

Angiotensin: Angiotensin I, consisting of 10 amino acids, has slight effect on blood pressure. Angiotensin II, consisting of 8 amino acids, has significant effect on blood pressure.

Insulin: It consists of 51 amino acids, contains two polypeptide chains linked together by two S-S bridges. This hormone helps in the utilization of sugar by the cells.

PROTEINS

The proteins are polymers of a large number of amino acids. However, their actual structure is not like a long chain, but is modified considerably by various forces, the most important of which is hydrogen bonding.

Forces which modify protein structure are:

a. **Hydrogen bond:** A hydrogen atom, joined to an electronegative element, when comes in the vicinity of another electronegative element of small atomic radius (N, O), it is attracted by the latter, and behaves as if it is shared by both electronegative elements. Hydrogen bonding is very common in proteins and nucleic acids. It is a weak ionic attraction but the reinforced action of several hydrogen bonds makes the structure very stable.

b. **Disulfide bond:** It is a covalent bond formed between two cysteine residues when they are in vicinity. It is a very stable bond. Insulin has both intrachain as well as interchain disulfide bonds.

c. **Ionic bond:** Ionic attraction between oppositely charged groups occurs when they are close. This is actually not a bond but is very weak attraction. The most common oppositely charged groups in a protein molecule are free COO^- of glutamic and aspartic acids and free NH_3^+ of lysine, arginine and histidine.

Under the influence of these forces, the protein structure is considerably modified and altered.

Protein Structure

The simplest description of protein structure is to write the sequence of amino acids in a polypeptide chain. This is called *primary* structure. The long polypeptide chain acquires coiled structure by means of mostly hydrogen bonds and occasionally disulfide bonds. This is known as *secondary* structure. The coiled proteins structure is further modified to assume folded structure. It is called the *tertiary* structure of proteins. The quaternary structure is observed in those proteins which are made up of two or more polypeptides. All these polypeptides combine together each having their primary, secondary and tertiary structure intact (Fig. 2.1).

Proteins made up of two or more polypeptide chains also have quaternary structure. An example is apoferritin. It has "ping-pong" ball structure. As many as 24 "ping-pong" balls put together will imitate apoferritin molecule in which each ball represents one polypeptide chain (Fig. 2.1). The vacant spaces between the balls allow the iron salts to enter and reside, thus converting apoferritin into ferritin.

Classification of Proteins

Like carbohydrates and lipids, proteins are classified into three major classes on the basis of products obtained on their hydrolysis (Table 2.1).

1. **Simple proteins:** Proteins which liberate only amino acids on their hydrolysis. Albumin and globulin present in blood plasma are well known examples. Other examples are basic proteins histones found in association with nucleic acids. Then there is scleroprotein which is totally insoluble.

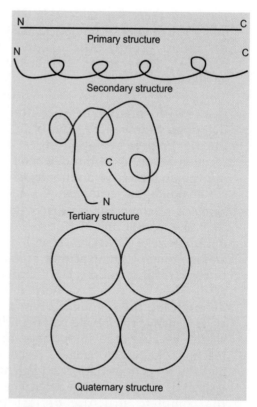

Fig. 2.1: Four levels of protein structure

2. **Conjugated proteins:** Those proteins which on complete hydrolysis, liberate a non-protein substance (prosthetic group), in addition to amino acids. The nucleoproteins are good examples of this class. These contain nucleic acid DNA or RNA united to a protein. The other common example is casein of milk which contains phosphate group.

3. **Derived proteins:** This group contains proteoses, polypeptides or peptides derived from above class of proteins. The examples are denatured proteins and products of partial hydrolysis of a native protein (as occurs in the gut).

PHYSICOCHEMICAL PROPERTIES OF PROTEINS

The proteins are high molecular compounds which exhibit characteristic properties in

Table 2.1: Classification of proteins

Class	Characteristics	Examples
Simple proteins		
a. Albumins	Soluble in water, coagulates by heat	Ovalbumin (egg), lactalbumin (milk)
b. Globulins	Insoluble in water, soluble in dilute salt solution	Vitellin (egg yolk), tuberin (Potato)
c. Glutelins	Insoluble in water, soluble in dilute acid and alkalis	Glutenin (wheat), oryzenin (rice)
d. Prolamines	Insoluble in water, soluble in 70% alcohol	Gliadin (wheat), zein (maize)
e. Protamines	Soluble in water, dilute acids and alkalis	Salmine (salmon sperm)
f. Histones	Soluble in water	Nucleohistone of the thymus gland
g. Scleroprotein	Totally insoluble	Keratin, collagen
Conjugated proteins		
a. Nucleoproteins	Consisting of simple protein and nucleic acids, soluble in water	Nucleohistones
b. Lipoproteins	Consisting of protein and lipids	Lipoprotein of plasma
c. Phosphoproteins	Protein containing phosphate	Caseinogen (milk), ovivitellin (egg yolk)
d. Chromoproteins	Consisting of protein and the colored compound (chromophore)	Haemoglobin, myoglobin
e. Metalloproteins	Protein containing metal ions	Ceruplasmin (Cu), ferritin (Fe)
f. Glycoproteins	Combination of protein with carbohydrates	Ovomucoid (egg white), mucin (saliva)
Derived proteins		
a. Primary derivatives		
1. Coagulated protein	Proteins coagulated by the action of heat, X-rays, UV rays, etc.	Coagulated albumin
b. Secondary derivatives		
1. Proteoses	Formed by the action of pepsin or trypsin, incoagulable by heat	Albumin proteose
2. Peptones	Formed by further hydrolysis of proteoses. Soluble in water, incoagulable by heat	Peptones
3. Peptides	Compounds containing two or more amino acids	Glycylalanine

different medium. Some of these properties are described here.

1. **Isoelectric pH:** Many ionizable groups are present in protein molecules. Depending on the pH of the medium, some of these groups act as proton donors and some other act as proton acceptors. Thus, proteins are amphoteric compounds. At a specific pH, the protein exists as a dipolar ion (one positive and negative ion) or zwitter ion, so at this pH the net charge of a protein becomes zero. This pH is known as isoelectric pH of the protein. The molecule having no net charge does not move in an electric field.

2. **Solubility:** Proteins behave differently in solution. Globular proteins are generally more soluble in aqueous medium in comparison to elongated fibrous proteins such as keratins. Solubility behavior of proteins, however, is influenced by the nature of solvent, pH, temperature, etc.

3. **Precipitation:** Proteins may be precipitated in three different ways as follows:

   a. *Isoelectric precipitation:* At isoelectric pH, a protein does not have any net charge. They easily aggregate and precipitate without denaturation due to minimum electrostatic repulsion.

   b. *Salting out:* Proteins in aqueous medium can be precipitated by adding trichloroacetic acid (TCA) or salts of heavy metals. Known as salting out and concentrated solution of neutral minerals salts, such as $MgSO_4$ and Na_2SO_4 are commonly used for this purpose.

   c. *Action of non-polar organic solvents:* A non-polar solvent-like chloroform enhances the electrostatic attraction between the ions of proteins and thus facilitates their aggregation and precipitation.

Functions of Proteins

Proteins perform a variety of functions. This can also be criteria of their classification (Table 2.2).

Importance of Proteins

Animal tissues are made up of proteins in contrast to plant tissues which are made up of carbohydrates. All enzymes and some hormones are proteins. In addition, proteins as nucleoproteins are concerned with heredity. Proteins also give energy by catabolism of amino acids. One gram of protein gives approximately 4 calories in the body, an amount equal to carbohydrates. Proteins are important constituents of foods because they form human tissues. Some common food sources (vegetarian and non-vegetarian) are shown in Fig. 2.2a and b, respectively.

Denaturation of Proteins

Denaturation is the most important property of proteins. The protein molecule

Table 2.2: Functions of proteins

Protein functions	Examples	Classes
1. To form structure of tissues	Collagen	Structural proteins
2. To function in contraction of muscles	Actin, myosin	Contractile proteins
3. To transport substances	Hemoglobin	Transport proteins
4. To catalyze chemical reactions	All enzymes	Catalytic proteins
5. To regulate metabolism	Protein hormones	Regulatory proteins
6. To transfer heritable characters	Nucleoproteins	Genetic proteins
7. To maintain immunity	Gamma globulins	Immunoproteins

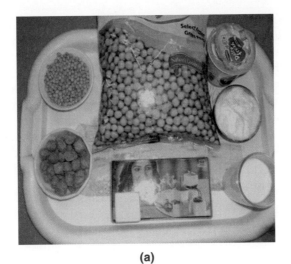

(a)

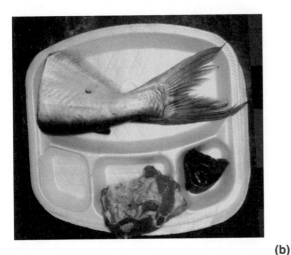
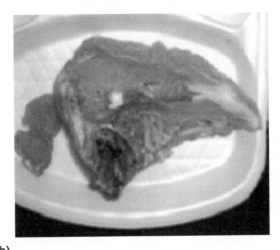

(b)

Fig. 2.2: (a) Vegetarian and (b) non-vegetarian proteins

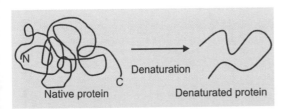

Fig. 2.3: Denaturation of protein

is very sensitive to its environmental conditions. Any change in conditions like temperature or pH will unfold the complex native structure of protein (Fig. 2.3) by breaking hydrogen bonds and other weak bonds but without hydrolyzing it. Denaturation actually results into change in the physical, physiological and immunological properties of the native proteins.

Causes of denaturation: Denaturation can be caused by mechanical, physical or chemical agents like grinding, heating or acids, respectively.

Effect of denaturation: Denaturation results into change of physical properties of proteins. The most conspicuous is solubility. Hence, denatured proteins are precipitated or coagulated. The chemical properties are not altered. The other change is in biological properties. If the protein is an enzyme, it will no longer exhibit enzymatic activity upon denaturation. The denatured protein differs from native protein in no more having extensive hydrogen bonding and cross links.

Advantages of denaturation:

1. Denaturation of food proteins make it more easily digestible by opening the folded molecule and exposing hidden peptide bonds. It occurs during cooking by application of heat and by HCl in the stomach.

2. Globular proteins on denaturation become elongated molecules which are used to form artificial fibers.

Chemistry of Lipids

3

INTRODUCTION

This group of compounds contains naturally occurring substances which differ from carbohydrates and proteins in being insoluble in water. The insolubility of lipids in water poses problems in their absorption and transport which are surmounted by special mechanisms. While the primary function of carbohydrates is to give energy, the function of proteins is mainly to form tissues. Lipids have dual function in the body—the major lipid, fat, gives energy to the body and is also part of tissues along with compound lipids–phospholipids and glycolipids.

DEFINITION

The lipids are a group of substances which are:

i. Insoluble in water
ii. Greasy in nature
iii. Esters of fatty acids or substances capable of forming such esters.

CLASSIFICATION

As for carbohydrates and proteins, lipids are classified into three classes on the basis of knowledge of products obtained on hydrolysis (Fig. 3.1).

Simple Lipids

These are esters of fatty acids with alcohols. The most common example is fats which are

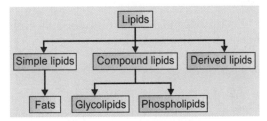

Fig. 3.1: Classification of lipids

esters of fatty acids with glycerol. Oils are those fats which are liquid at ordinary room temperature.

Compound Lipids

These are esters of fatty acids with alcohols, but also contain some other group, the natures of which are used to sub-classify them. For example, phospholipids, gly-colipids.

a. Phospholipids

These contain two fatty acids and one ortho phosphoric acid molecule combined to glycerol. A nitrogen containing compound is also bound to phosphoric acid. The phospholipids can be represented as:

CH₂OH	CH₂O–fatty acid
CHOH	CHO–fatty acid
CH₂OH	CH₂O–phosphoric acid–N base
Glycerol	Phospholipid

Or simply: Fatty acids (2)—glycerol–phosphoric acid–N base.

Phospholipids are further classified on the basis of N base. Examples are lecithin and cephalin which contains choline and ethanolamine, respectively, as nitrogenous base. Another member, sphingomyelins, contains one fatty acid, phosphoric acid and choline or ethanolamine but glycerol is replaced by an amino alcohol—sphingol or sphingosine.

Fatty acid (1)—sphingol-phosphoric acid-choline or ethanolamine.

Lecithin is most important phospholipid, hence, it is discussed here.

Lecithin (Fig. 3.2)

- Lecithin is very important phospholipid. Dietary lecithin reduces deposition of fat in liver and thus prevents development of fatty liver, so it is a lipotropic factor.
- The snake venom hydrolyzes β-carbon of lecithin and form lysolecithin which hemolyzes the erythrocytes.
- Lecithin is present in lung alveoli to reduce the surface tension and prevent the collapse of alveolus. In certain new-born infants, lecithin is lacking so they suffer from this problem. This causes difficulty in respiration (Fig. 3.3). This condition is called respiratory distress syndrome (RDS).

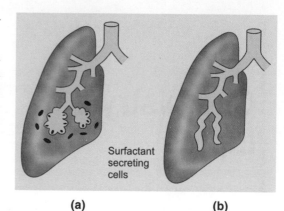

Surfactant secreting cells

(a)   **(b)**

Fig. 3.3: (a) Normal expansion of alveoli due to normal secretion of surfactant (lecithin) and **(b)** failure of alveoli to expand due to lack of surfactant (lecithin)

b. Glycolipids

These contain fatty acid, an alcohol (sphingol) and a carbohydrate, which is either glucose or galactose, hence, these are called glycolipids. These are also known as cerebrosides as they are mainly present in brain and myelin sheath of nerves. Glycolipids can be represented as:

Fatty acid–sphingol–carbohydrate

Derived Lipids

These are substances derived from above groups by hydrolysis. Important derived lipids are fatty acids and alcohols. This group includes fatty acids, alcohols, steroids and fat soluble vitamins A, D, E and K.

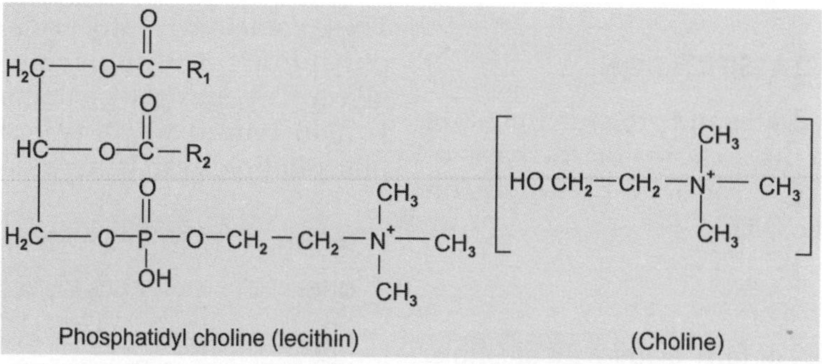

Phosphatidyl choline (lecithin)   (Choline)

Fig. 3.2: Structure of phospholipid (lecithin)

FATTY ACIDS

Fatty acids most commonly found in fats and other lipids are straight chain compounds with even number of carbon atoms. They may be saturated or unsaturated.

Saturated fatty acids: The general formula of saturated fatty acids is $C_nH_{2n+1}.COOH$. It has a polar end with a free –COOH group and non-polar end with hydrocarbon chain. Fatty acids with less carbon atoms are readily miscible with water and the solubility decreases with increase in carbon atoms. Saturated fatty acids with less than 10 carbon atoms are liquid at room temperature and those having more are solids. Melting point of these fatty acids increase with increase in number of carbon atoms. A number of saturated fatty acids are there in nature starting from acetic acid (Table 3.1).

Unsaturated fatty acids: Unsaturated fatty acids having two or more double bonds are called polyunsaturated fatty acids (PUFA) while those with only one double bond are called monounsaturated fatty acids (MUFA). Unsaturated fatty acids show several forms of different isomerisms. The fatty acids with same molecular formula as well as same number of double bond may differ in the location of double bonds exhibiting positional isomerism. Oleic acid has 15 different positional isomerisms. Again the orientation of the two hydrogen atoms attached to the two carbon atoms joined by the double bonds may differ, giving rise to geometric isomerism. If the hydrogen atoms are placed on the same side of the double bond, cis-isomer results but if these are placed on either side of the double bond, it is trans-isomer. An example of cis-trans-isomerism has shown in Fig. 3.4.

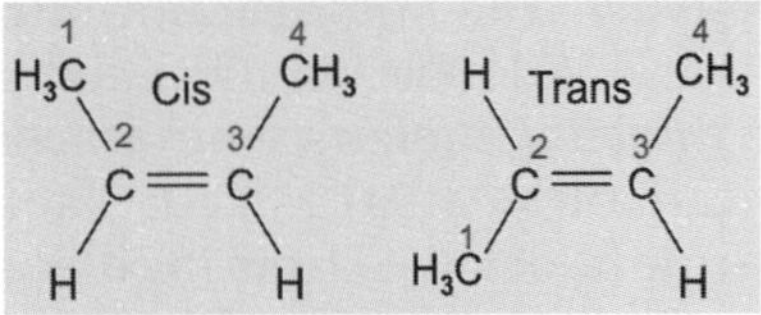

Fig. 3.4: Cis- and trans-isomers

Carbon atoms of fatty acids are numbered from carboxyl carbon. Various conventions are used to indicate the position of double bonds in the fatty acid molecules. Like Δ^9 indicates a double bond between carbon atoms 9 and 10 of the fatty acid.

The Greek alphabets (α, β, γ,...., ω) are used to identify the location of the double bonds. The "alpha" carbon is the carbon next to the carboxyl group and "omega" is the last letter of the Greek alphabet. Linoleic

---

Table 3.1: Naturally occurring common saturated fatty acids and their sources

Common names	Molecular formulae	Food sources
Butyric acid	$C_3H_7.COOH$	Butter
Caproic acid	$C_5H_{11}.COOH$	Butter
Caprylic acid	$C_7H_{15}.COOH$	Fats of plant origin
Capric acid	$C_9H_{19}.COOH$	Fats of plant origin
Lauric acid	$C_{11}H_{23}.COOH$	Palm kernels, cinnamon, coconut oil
Myristic acid	$C_{13}H_{27}.COOH$	Nutmeg, palm kernels, coconut oil
Palmitic acid	$C_{15}H_{31}.COOH$	Palm oil, animal and plant fat
Stearic acid	$C_{17}H_{35}.COOH$	Animal fat and plant oil
Arachidic acid	$C_{19}H_{39}.COOH$	Groundnut oil
Lignoceric acid	$C_{23}H_{47}.COOH$	Groundnut oil

acid is an omega-6-fatty acid because it has a double bond six carbons away from the "omega" carbon. Similarly, alpha-linoleic acid is an "omega-3 fatty acid because it has a double bond three carbons away from the "omega" carbon.

Some commonly occurring unsaturated fatty acids are shown in Table 3.2.

Important members are oleic acid (C_{18}), linoleic acid (C_{18}), linolenic acid (C_{18}) and arachidonic acid (C_{20}) which contain one, two, three and four double bonds, respectively. The body cannot introduce more than one double bond in a compound, hence linoleic, linolenic and arachidonic acids cannot be synthesized. Therefore, these are to be obtained from the diet and are called essential fatty acids. They have some important functions in the body, hence, their deficiency causes disease.

Essential fatty acids: Rats fed on a purified non-lipid diet to which vitamin A and D were added exhibited reduced growth rate, reproductive deficiency, scaly skin, necrosis of the tail and lesion in the urinary system which was found to be cured by the addition of these fatty acids. However, their deficiency in man has not been demonstrated unequivocally.

The polyunsaturated fatty acid (PUFA) content of some fats and oils is given in Table 3.3.

Table 3.3: PUFA content of some fats and oils

Fats and oils	PUFA (%)
Butter fat	3.6
Coconut oil	1.5
Vanaspati ghee	3.0
Ghee	2.6
Groundnut oil	21.8
Sesame oil	43.7
Cotton seed oil	47.8
Soybean oil	50.7
Corn oil	56.3
Sunflower oil	68.0
Safflower oil	78.0

Our PUFA requirements can be met by daily consumption of 15–25 gm of appropriate lipids.

The function of the essential fatty acids appears to be numerous, although not well defined. They are found in the structural lipids of the cell, are concerned with the structural integrity of the mitochondrial membrane, and occur in high concentration in the reproductive organs. In many of their structural functions, essential fatty acids are present as phospholipids, most frequently, the β-position is occupied by an unsaturated fatty acid (and often the α-position as well). There, they have a role in the metabolism of

Table 3.2: Naturally occuring common unsaturated fatty acids

Common names	Chemical structures	Food sources
Palmitoleic acid	$CH_3(CH_2)_5CH=CH(CH_2)_7COOH$	All fats
Oleic acid	$CH_3(CH_2)_7CH=CH(CH_2)_7COOH$	All fats, abundant in olive oil
Elaidic acid	$CH_3(CH_2)_7CH=CH(CH_2)_7COOH$	Hydrogenated fat, margarine
Linoleic acid	$CH_3(CH_2)_4CH=CH(CH_2)_7COOH$	Mainly vegetables oils, particularly linseed oil
Linolenic acid	$CH_3CH_2CH=CHCH_2CH=CHCH_2CH=CH-(CH_2)_7COOH$	Mainly vegetables oils, particularly linseed oil
Arachidonic acid	$CH_3(CH_2)_4CH=CHCH_2CH=CHCH_2-CH=CHCH_2CH=CH(CH_2)_3COOH$	Peanut oil, groundnut oil, traces in some animal fats

cholesterol, i.e. possibly cholesterol esters of polyunsaturated fatty acids are more rapidly metabolized by the liver and other tissues for excretion. Arachidonic acid is the precursor of prostaglandins which might explain some deficiency symptoms and essentiality of PUFA or essential fatty acids.

CHEMICAL PROPERTIES OF FATTY ACIDS

- **Esterification:** Like any other organic acids, fatty acids form esters with various alcohols. The mono, di- and tri-acyl glycerols are esters of glycerol with one, two and three fatty acids, respectively.
- **Soap formation:** When fatty acids react with alkalis, salts of fatty acids are formed commonly called as 'SOAPS'. Potassium soap of fatty acids is more water soluble than sodium soap.
- **Hydrogenation:** When exposed to hydrogen at high temperature in presence of nickel and platinum catalyst, unsaturated fatty acids (containing double bonds) accept hydrogen at the double bonds and are converted to a saturated fatty acid (Fig. 3.5).

$$-C = C- \ + \ H_2 \ \xrightarrow[\text{High temp}]{\text{Ni}} \ -CH - CH-$$

Fig. 3.5: Hydrogenation reaction

Hydrogenation is used to change liquid oil into a semi-solid or solid fat at ambient temperature to enhance oxidative stability.

- **Halogenation:** Fatty acid accepts chlorine and iodine at the double bonds when reacted with reagents, such as iodine monochloride and fatty halide results.

FATS

Fats are quantitatively most significant lipids in the body and the diet. These contain glycerol esterified with fatty acids. Glycerol has three alcoholic groups, so it can combine with one, two or three fatty acids giving rise to monoglyceride, diglyceride and triglyceride, respectively (Fig. 3.6). Triglycerides are also known as neutral fats. Some common dietary fats and oils are shown in Fig. 3.7.

The different vegetable oils and animal fats are chemically triglycerides. They differ in their fatty acid composition. Oils are rich in unsaturated fatty acids.

Margarine is extensively used as a cheap substitute of butter. The word margarine is derived from the Greek margarine (pearl), as fat when churned with milk produces globule resembling pearls. Margarine is prepared from vegetables oils, such as coconut, groundnut and soybean. The heated oil is being churned with skimmed milk. Yellow color is added to make the margarine look like butter.

Physical Properties of Fats

1. Fats are colorless, tasteless and odorless. The color, odor and taste of natural oils and fat is due to other substances dissolved in them.
2. **Emulsification:** The dispersion of one liquid into another is called an emulsion. This is a colloidal solution. Generally oil and water do not mix. They are immiscible. However, in presence of certain substances (like soap or bile salts), tiny globules of oil get dispersed in water. This dispersion is called an emulsion and the substances are called emulsifying agents. These agents lower the surface tension of water and thus facilitate mixing of two liquids. Because of this property, emulsifying agents are used as detergents to wash clothes and clean utensils of oil, grease and adhering dirt.

Chemical Properties of Fats

1. **Hydrolysis:** Fats being esters can be hydrolyzed. The hydrolysis may be

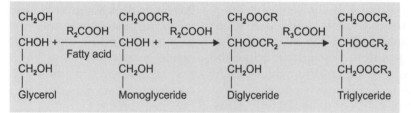

Fig. 3.6: Formation of glycerides

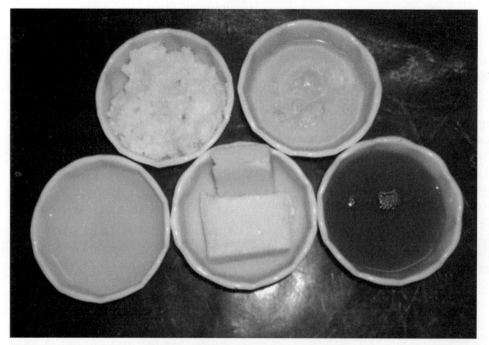

Fig. 3.7: Food sources of fats and oils

brought about by an acid, alkali or enzyme (lipase in the gut). The complete hydrolysis of a fat liberates three fatty acid molecules and a glycerol. Partial hydrolysis librates fatty acids and mono- or diglycerides.

Fat + Water ⇌ Glycerol +
3 Fatty acids

2. **Saponification:** Hydrolysis of a fat by alkali is called saponification. The products of hydrolysis are glycerol and alkali salt of the fatty acids called soap (Fig. 3.8). This is the method by which soap is manufactured. Glycerol is produced as a byproduct of this reaction which is removed. If some glycerol is allowed to remain in soap, it becomes transparent and is much soothing to the skin.

3. **Rancidity:** It is the spoilage of edible fat due to formation of peroxides and per-acids by the action of heat, air and humidity on unsaturated bonds in a fat. Rancid fat is unpalatable, slightly toxic and destructive to carotene and vitamins.

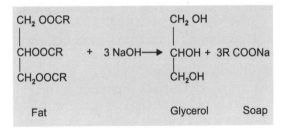

Fig. 3.8: Saponification

Certain substances, like vitamin E, retard the development of rancidity in fats and oils. These are called anti-oxidants. On the other hand, pro-oxidants are the substances which increase the susceptibility of fats to oxidation, for example, Cu^{2+}, Fe^{3+} ions act as pro-oxidants. In Indian households, housewives generally have a practice to save remaining oil or fat after frying for use some days later. This may cause the fat or oil to become rancid. It is harmful, hence, this practice should be stopped.

4. **Unsaturation reactions:** Unsaturated bonds in a fat undergo addition reactions. They can accept hydrogen, oxygen or iodine. In hydrogenation of fat, an unsaturated fat is made to react with hydrogen at high temperature in presence of a metal, like nickel, as a catalyst. This is how vanaspati ghee is manufactured. The hydrogenated fat has higher melting point, is harder and there is no danger of its spoilage due to rancidity.

Characterization of Fats

Different fats and oils have similar physical properties. In order to identify them, certain chemical parameters are to be determined. Two such parameters are:

1. **Saponificaton number:** It is the number of mg of KOH required to completely saponify 1 g of fat or oil. It varies inversely with the molecular weight of the fat and is a measure of mean molecular weight of fatty acids present in the fat.

2. **Iodine number:** It is the number of mg of iodine absorbed by 1 g of fat and is the measure of the degree of unsaturation of the fat.

STEROIDS

Natural fat usually contains minute amount of other greasy substances, which occur as "unsaponifiable residue". The steroids are an example of such compounds. All the steroids have a similar cyclic nucleus resembling phenanthrene (three six-membered rings A, B and C fused together) to which a five membered cyclopentane ring D is attached. The rings are completely saturated, so the parent substance is better designated as "cyclopentanoperhydrophenanthrene" (Fig. 3.9).

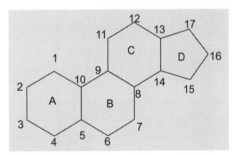

Fig. 3.9: Cyclopentanoperhydrophenanthrene nucleus

Methyl groups are frequently attached at positions 10 and 13. A side chain at position 17 is usually found. Similarly, an oxygen containing group is present at position no. 3.

Cholesterol is the most important compound of this class (Fig. 3.10). It is widely

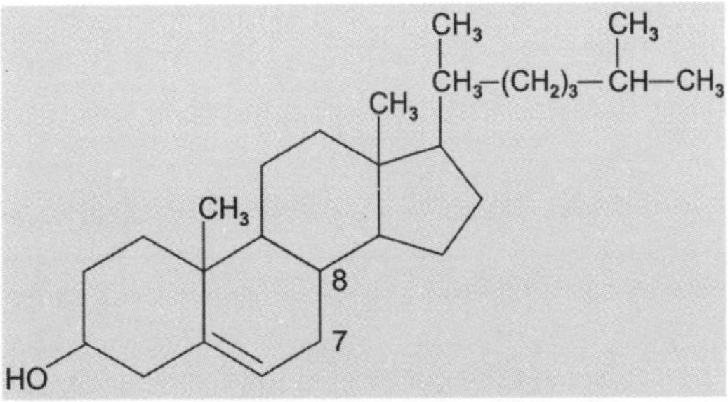

Fig. 3.10: Cholesterol

distributed in all cells of the body, but particularly in nervous tissue. It occurs in animal fats but not in plant fats. Animal tissues are capable of synthesizing cholesterol. All other steroids are then derived from cholesterol. These include bile acids, steroids, hormones (male and female sex hormones, adrenocortical hormones, progesterone from corpus luteum) and bile acids.

Steroids are of many types. These are given below:

a. Sterols: Cholesterol, ergosterol

b. Bile acids: Glycocholic acid, taurocholic acid

c. Hormones: Testosterone, estradiol, corticosterone

d. Vitamin: Vitamin D_2 and D_3

e. Cardiac glycosides: Digitonin

Sterols of vegetables origin are called "phytosterols". They have the same basic structure as cholesterol, but differ in side chain attached to carbon 17, phytosterol, such as stigmasterol from soybean oil, are of current interest because they lower blood cholesterol levels.

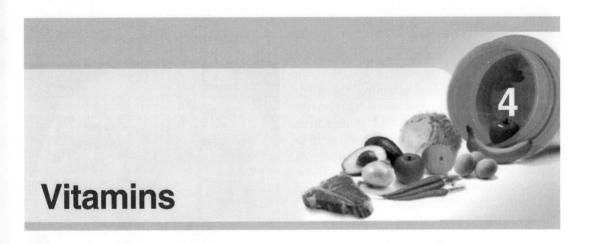

Vitamins

INTRODUCTION

In addition to carbohydrates, proteins, fats and mineral salts, animals require a diverse group of compounds for growth and maintenance of body. This realization has resulted into discovery of several essential nutrients in the 19th and 20th century. These were considered the "protective food".

DEFINITION

In the simple words, "Vitamins are described as organic compounds, required in minute amounts in the diet for normal growth and maintenance of life." Their deficiency results into specific changes in the structure or function of the body which is described as 'deficiency disease' and which is usually corrected by administration of missing nutrient/vitamin.

CLASSIFICATION

In the beginning, as different vitamins were discovered, their chemical structures were not known, hence, they were designated by letters of the alphabet, viz. A, C, B_1, B_2, etc. and classified on the basis of solubility as fat soluble and water soluble. Now the chemical structure is well established, so chemical names have also been given to them. However, this classification is still retained as many similarities exist within the group and there are many differences between the two groups.

There are four fat soluble vitamins—vitamin A, D, E and K. Their absorption requires bile salts, so deficiency develops in conditions associated with impaired secretion of bile. They are stored to a considerable extent in the body so it takes much longer to develop the deficiency disease. The vitamin activity is exhibited by more than one chemical compound. They all have a typical nuclear structure with a long side chain.

On the other hand, there are several members of water soluble vitamins—thiamine, riboflavin, niacin, pyridoxal, biotin, folic acid, vitamin B_{12}, and pantothenic acid (collectively grouped as B-complex vitamins) and vitamin C or ascorbic acid. Members of this group of vitamins are not stored in the body to any appreciable extent, hence, the deficiency develops very quickly. The vitamin activity is shown by a single molecular species. Many of these vitamins are synthesized by intestinal bacteria, a part of which is available to host organism. Therefore, vitamin deficiency usually develops on antibiotic therapy if continued for long time. The vitamins of B-complex group are known to act as coenzymes of specific enzymes, so enzyme activity is reduced in that particular vitamin deficiency, thus, affecting the relevant chemical reaction.

Provitamins

Apart from established vitamins, there are instances of some compounds which do not exert vitamin activity as such but are active only after chemical transformation into other compound. The example is β-carotene, which forms vitamin A in the body. These are known as previtamins or precursor of vitamins or provitamins.

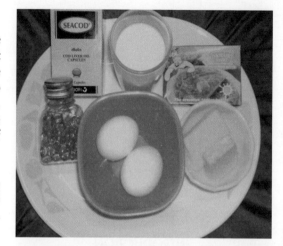

FAT SOLUBLE VITAMINS

There are four fat soluble vitamins— vitamins A, D, E and K.

VITAMIN A

Introduction

It is also known as anti-infective factor. Its chemical name is retinol as it is an alcohol and is present in retina for vision.

The molecular formula is $C_{20}H_{30}O$ or $C_{20}H_{29}OH$. It has a β-ionone ring and a primary alcoholic group (CH_2OH) in the side chain. The alcoholic group (–OH) is easily oxidized into aldehyde group (–CHO) known as retinal or retinine or vitamin A_1 aldehyde and further into retinoic acid (–COOH).

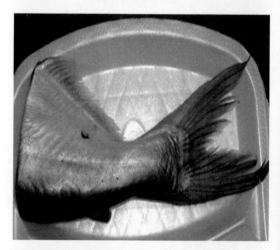

Food Sources

Vitamin A is obtained in the diet as preformed vitamin or from its precursors, known as provitamins. Preformed vitamin is exclusively found in animal food. Richest source is fish liver oil. Other good sources are fish, liver, eggs, milk and butter (Fig. 4.1a). Provitamins are confined to vegetable food. Plant pigments like carotene are converted to vitamin A in the body. Best source is carrots. Main sources are green leafy vegetables and fruits like, spinach, pumpkin, sweet potatoes, papaya and tomatoes (Fig. 4.1b). In general, pigmented vegetables and fruits, especially the yellow ones, contain large amount of β-carotene.

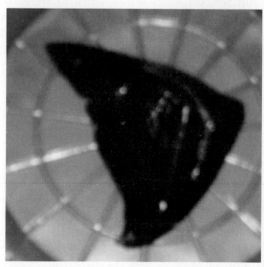

Fig. 4.1a: Food sources of vitamin A

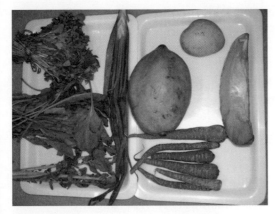

Fig. 4.1b: Food sources of provitamin A (carotene)

Dried fruits are concentrated sources. Loss of vitamin A during cooking is small.

Functions

All the three forms—retinol, retinal and retinoic acids have physiological functions in the body.

Retinol: It is essential for normal growth and reproduction. Vitamin A is considered as an important growth factor.

Retinal: It is concerned with and is essential for vision. The human retina contains photoreceptor cells called rods, which contain conjugated protein rhodopsin, made of protein opsin and retinal (vitamin A aldehyde). Actually 11-cis-isomer of retinal is present.

Retinoic acid: It is essential for formation of glycoproteins and thus for epithelial cells.

Deficiency

Most of the deficiency symptoms are explained on the basis of the role of vitamin A in structure and function of epithelium, growth and vision.

a. *Epithelium:* Vitamin A is essential for normal structure and function of epithelial tissues, e.g. respiratory tract, urinary tract, digestive tract, cornea, etc.

In its absence, normal secretory epithelium is replaced by dry keratinized epithelium which is more susceptible to invasion by infectious organisms.

b. *Growth:* Vitamin A is a growth factor. Growth retardation is observed in experimental animals in vitamin A deficiency. The skeleton is affected first and then the soft tissues are involved. Collagenous tissues are particularly affected. The mucopolysaccharide (ground substance) synthesis is reduced which is restored to normal when the vitamin is provided.

c. *Eye and Vision:*

(i) *Eye:* Various changes that occur in vitamin A deficiency in eyes are:

• *Bitot's spots*: White opaque spots in conjunctiva (Fig. 4.2).

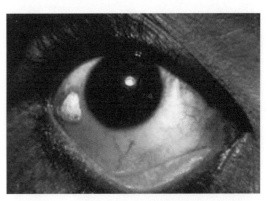

Fig. 4.2: Bitot's spot

• *Xerosis*: Dry conjunctiva, hazy wrinkled cornea (Fig. 4.3).

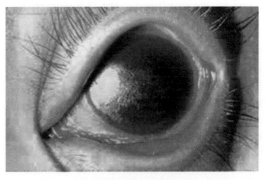

Fig. 4.3: Xerosis

- *Xerophthalmia: Dry eyes*—Dryness, thickening and loss of transparency of ocular tissue (Blindness) (Fig. 4.4).

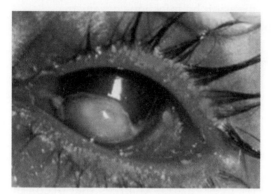

Fig. 4.4: Xerophthalmia

- *Keratomalacia:* Keratinization of corneal epithelium (softening and ulceration) (Fig. 4.5).

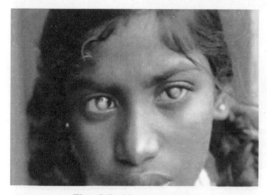

Fig. 4.5: Keratomalacia

(ii) *Vision:* Vitamin A deficiency leads to night blindness. Night blindness is inability to see in the subdued light. The reactions occurring in retina during the visual process are shown in Wald cycle or rhodopsin cycle (Fig. 4.6).

Under normal conditions, in the retina of the eye, the rate of breakdown of rhodopsin is equalled by the rate of regeneration. In vitamin A deficiency, the rate of regeneration is retarded because of shortage of precursor substances. This results in night blindness or nyctalopia. A night blind individual takes much longer to regenerate his visual purple or rhodopsin when passing from bright light to dim light.

Requirement

Adults require 5,000 IU of vitamin A while increased requirement is suggested in pregnancy (6,000 IU) and lactation (8,000 IU). Children should take 2,000–5,000 IU as per their age.

Toxicity

Hypervitaminosis A: Therapeutic doses of vitamin A in excess of 50,000 IU daily over prolonged periods may be toxic to adults. Lesser doses will produce symptoms in children. The common symptoms of toxicity are anorexia, hyperirritability, and drying and desquamation of the skin. Loss of hair, bone and joint pain, bone fragility, headache, and enlargement of the liver and spleen are quite frequent.

VITAMIN D

Introduction

Vitamin D prevents rickets, hence, it is called anti-rachitic factor. Chemically it is known as calciferol because of its role in calcium metabolism.

Vitamins D are a group of sterol compounds. Two forms of vitamin D are well known—vitamin D_2 or ergocalciferol and vitamin D_3 or cholecalciferol. These are found in plants and animals, respectively.

Food Sources

The best source is cod liver oil and other fish liver oils. Mention should be made of the cheapest source which is sunlight induced synthesis of vitamin D_3 in skin. The major natural food sources are fish, liver oils, egg yolk and liver (Fig. 4.7). Endogenous production is the most important source. The content in milk is low, yet rickets only occurs when milk is not given and sunshine is not available. Thus, vitamin D in milk may

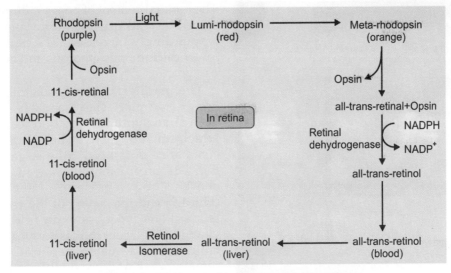

Fig. 4.6: Wald cycle (rhodopsin cycle) in retina

be more biologically available than from other dietary sources.

Functions

The vitamin D is mainly concerned with metabolism of calcium. The principal action of vitamin D is to increase the calcium absorption from intestine. It is also concerned with intestinal absorption, renal reabsorption and bone mobilization of calcium. In all these functions, dietary vitamin D is effective only after its conversion in the body into active form (1, 25-dihydroxycholecalciferol). It also has a role in tubular reabsorption of phosphate (and of calcium) by kidney. Thus, it maintains a proper concentration of calcium and phosphorous in the blood. The ideal Calcium × Phosphorous ratio is 50 in children and 40 in adults; a ratio below 30 leads to rickets (normal serum calcium level is 9 to 11.5 mg% and inorganic phosphorous in children is 4 to 7 mg% and 3 to 6 mg% in adults.

The vitamin D has a direct effect on calcification process. Administration of vitamin D to animals deficient in the vitamin increases the rate of deposition and reabsorption of minerals from bone. It is claimed that vitamin D help in deposition of crystalline, rather than amorphous calcium phosphate in bones by supplying calcium and phosphate in proper concentration to the bony matrix. The crystalline structure makes the bones stronger.

Sunlight and Vitamin D Requirements

The dietary requirement of vitamin D depends a lot on its synthesis by the body. The exposure of unprotected skin to two sessions of 15 minutes of sunlight each week will produce adequate amounts of vitamin D. If the body cannot produce enough vitamin D because of insufficient sunlight exposure, it will need to obtain it from foods and perhaps supplements.

Deficiency

Deficiency of vitamin D produces rickets in children and osteomalacia in adults. These conditions are due to either dietary inadequacy or malabsorption of vitamin D or insufficient exposure to sunlight (due to *Purdah* system).

Rickets: Rickets is a disease of infancy or early childhood, characterized by faulty deposition of calcium phosphate, with the result that the bones do not grow normally.

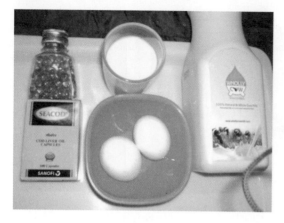

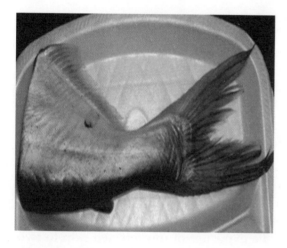

The mineral content of bones is diminished, the water and organic matter being correspondingly increased. The bones have lower calcium, phosphorous and carbonate content.

The manifestation of rickets includes bony deformities. The essential bony lesion is an abundant formation of osteoid tissue which fails to calcify. The characteristic signs are: "boss head" (the large head in Fig. 4.8), protrusion of forehead, "pigeon chest", "bow legs" and "knock knee" (Fig. 4.9) and thickening of the wrists and ankles. The most common finding in a vitamin D deficient child is bow legs. Due to faulty and inadequate mineralization, bones remain weak and are unable to bear the weight of the child and it bends.

Osteomalacia: Literally osteomalacia means softening of bones ('Osteo' stands for bones and 'malacia' means softening). It occurs mainly in women due to poor diet, low intake of milk, malabsorption of calcium (vitamin D deficiency due to purdah), repeated pregnancy and prolonged lactation. Clinically osteomalacia manifests as a skeletal pain, bony tenderness and fractures.

Requirement

WHO recommends 100 IU in adults and 400 IU to newborns and women during pregnancy and lactation.

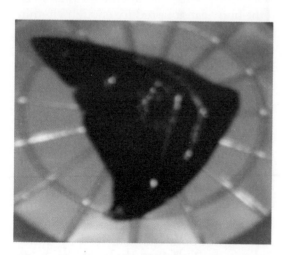

Fig. 4.7: Sources of vitamin D

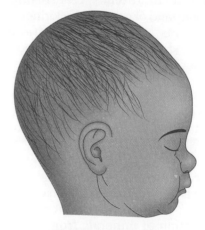

Fig. 4.8: Boss head

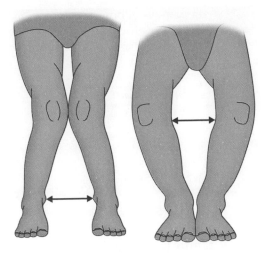

Fig. 4.9: Knock knee and bow legs

Hypervitaminosis D: The daily doses ranging from 1,000–3,000 IU are toxic. The symptoms of toxicity include nausea, diarrhea, weight loss, polyuria and nocturia.

VITAMIN E

Introduction

Chemically vitamin E is known as tocopherol also called anti-sterility factor because of earlier reports of sterility in animals on vitamin E deficiency. Hence, compounds possessing vitamin E activity are known as tocopherols. They are methylated derivatives of parent compound tocol (benzene and pyran rings fused together with an isoprenoid side chain). There are three isomers: α-tocopherol, β-tocopherol and γ-tocopherol; the first one is most active.

Food Sources

Vitamin E is found in lipids of green leafy plants and in oils of seeds. Wheat germ oil is the richest source. Cotton seed, corn and soybean oils are other good sources. Animal sources containing the highest amounts include eggs, liver and muscles meat (Fig. 4.10).

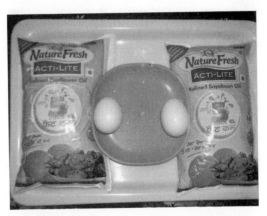

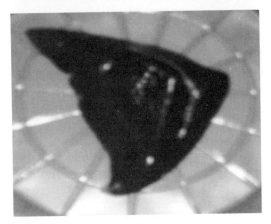

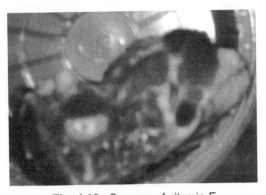

Fig. 4.10: Sources of vitamin E

Functions

Earlier vitamin E was called anti-sterility factor because the deficiency of vitamin E in rats and some other animals caused resorption of the fetus in the female and in the male, atrophy of spermatogenic tissue and permanent sterility was observed. There is no evidence of such an effect in humans. Nowadays, it is used mainly for its anti-oxidant function. It is the only physiological fat soluble, powerful anti-oxidant inhibiting oxidation of fats, carotene and vitamin A and probably thiol groups.

Requirement

An average adult requires 10–30 mg per day. This amount is easily supplied by diet, so deficiency is not seen.

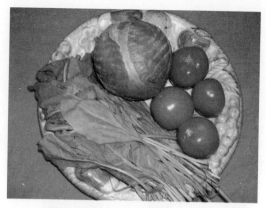

Fig. 4.11: Sources of Vitamin K

VITAMIN K

Introduction

This vitamin is called anti-hemorrhagic factor, as its deficiency produced uncontrolled hemorrhages due to defect in blood coagulation.

A number of chemical compounds which are related to 2-methyl-1, 4 naphthoquinone possess some degree of vitamin K activity. There are three compounds with vitamin K activity–K_1, K_2 and K_3. The structure of vitamin K resembles coenzyme Q.

Food Sources

The best dietary sources are green leafy vegetables. The vitamin is associated with chloroplast and bioavailability is variable. Spinach, cabbage and tomatoes are good sources (Fig. 4.11). Some vitamin K in the body is derived from gut bacteria, but this is poorly absorbed.

Functions

The best known function of vitamin K is to catalyze the synthesis of prothrombin by the liver. Vitamin K is also essential for the synthesis of some other coagulation factors. On injury, prothrombin is converted into active enzyme thrombin, which converts fibrinogen into the clot (fibrin). The clot acts as a physical barrier for further flow of blood (Fig. 4.12).

Vitamin K deficiency may occur following antibiotic therapy. Its deficiency may also occur in biliary obstruction or on administration of antagonist, dicoumarol. In vitamin K deficiency, clotting time of blood is increased.

WATER SOLUBLE VITAMINS

Vitamin C and B complex vitamins are soluble in water.

VITAMIN C (ASCORBIC ACID)

Introduction

Vitamin C is the oldest known vitamin. Chemically it is known as ascorbic acid,

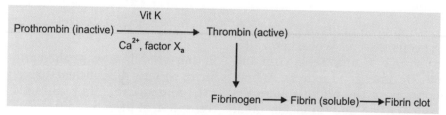

Fig. 4.12: Schematic of blood coagulation

hexuronic acid and cevitamic acid or anti-scorbutic vitamin as it cures scurvy.

Molecular formula of ascorbic acid is $C_6H_8O_6$. Its structure resembles hexoses, but it belongs to L-sugars which are not found in the body. It is a very strong reducing agent, thus it is a water soluble antioxidant. It is easily oxidized to dehydroascorbic acid. The acidic property of vitamin C is due to easy dissociation of two enolic groups.

Food Sources

Vitamin C is present in high concentration in green vegetables and citrus fruits, but the content is quite variable. Grains and nuts contain no vitamin C. Outstanding source is Amla (goose berry). Citrus fruits (oranges, lemons and grape fruits), tomatoes and other fresh fruits and vegetables are good sources (Fig. 4.13). The vitamin is easily destroyed by cooking since it is readily oxidized by air especially in alkaline medium and in presence of Cu^{++} ions or lost by cooking water.

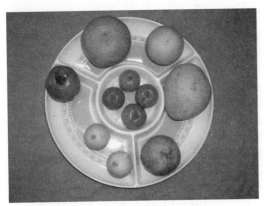

Fig. 4.13: Sources of vitamin C

Functions

Most important biochemical functions of vitamin C are the formation of intercellular cement substance and iron metabolism.

1. *Formation of intercellular substance:* Vitamin C is concerned fundamentally with the formation of intercellular cement substance of cartilage, dentin, bone and collagen. Vitamin C has a special role in collagen synthesis. Collagen is rich in hydroxyproline (12%) which is formed from proline by proline hydroxylase in presence of vitamin C. Hydroxylation actually involves the prolyl residues of the collagen precursor. Many of important clinical manifestations of vitamin C deficiency are directly due to abnormal structures of these.

2. *Iron absorption:* The vitamin C helps in the absorption of iron from gut and possibly in the utilization of iron as well. This is due to its reducing action as iron absorption occurs in ferrous state. Hypochromic, microcytic anemia sometimes occurring in scurvy can be explained on the basis of impaired metabolism of iron.

Deficiency

Severe vitamin C deficiency produces scurvy. Scurvy is characterized by failure in the formation and maintenance of intercellular materials, which in turn causes typical symptoms, such as hemorrhages, loosening of the teeth, poor wound healing and the easy fracturability of the bones.

Requirement

ICMR has suggested an intake of 40 mg/day for children and adults, more in pregnancy, double in lactation and half this amount in infants.

Toxicity

High doses of ascorbic acid have been reported to cause diarrhea and dry mouth and to promote renal stone formation, due in part to increased oxalate excretion and urinary acidification.

B COMPLEX VITAMINS

The B-series or B-complex vitamins are a group of water-soluble compounds, which have similar distribution in food and all are extractable in water, so generally their deficiency occur simultaneously rather than singly.

The following are generally accepted as B-vitamins: thiamine, riboflavin, niacin, pyridoxal, biotin, pantothenic acid, folic acid, vitamin B_{12} and lipoic acid. There is no agreement about the inclusion in this category of inositol, choline and p-amino-benzoic acid. A number of these compounds form coenzymes, which are mainly concerned with energy release in cellular oxidations or with protein synthesis. It is, therefore, not surprising that B-vitamin deficiencies should often manifest them-selves as a disorder of tissues in which rapid growth takes place even in the adults, namely, skin, mucous epithelium, digestive glands and bone marrow. Those tissues with high rates of metabolism including plant seeds are good source.

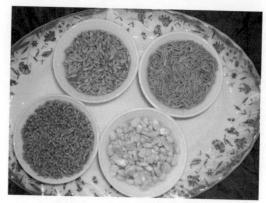

Fig. 4.14: Sources of vitamin B_1

THIAMINE (VITAMIN B₁)

Introduction

Vitamin B_1 is chemically known as thiamine. It is also called aneurine and anti beriberi factor. Thiamine contains two ring systems—a pyrimidine and a thiazole ring joined by a single carbon atom. It is a basic substance, hence, generally prepared as a salt chloride hydrochloride. The coenzyme form of vitamin is TPP or thiamine pyrophosphate. TPP requires Mg^{++} ions as activator.

Food Sources

All plant and animal tissues contain thiamine but in small amounts. More abundant sources are unrefined cereal grain, beans, nuts, meat (Fig. 4.14). Since this vitamin is water soluble and somewhat heat labile, it may be lost in cooking water. The small quantity required is easily provided if it is not removed during processing grains or destroyed during heating. Since it is water soluble, much of the vitamin is extracted in cooking liquid.

Functions

Thiamine coenzyme, TPP, catalyzes some very important reactions in carbohydrate metabolism. In humans, it catalyzes the oxidative decarboxylation of pyruvic and alpha-ketoglutaric acid (citric acid cycle) and transketolation reactions (hexose monophosphate pathway). Therefore, reactions are impaired in B_1 deficiency with the result that lactic and pyruvic acids accumulate in plasma and pentose sugars in RBCs in B_1 deficiency.

Deficiency

Biochemical role of thiamine are confined to carbohydrate metabolism. Therefore, signs of thiamine deficiency appear in people whose caloric (or carbohydrate) intake is disproportionately high as compared to their thiamine intake. Such an imbalance occurs endemically in certain areas of Asia where people subsist largely on polished, milled rice (the processing of which removes the thiamine) and also in chronic alcoholics who eat little food (alcoholic beverages provide calories but not thiamine).

Vitamin B_1 deficiency disease in humans is known as "beriberi", which affects cardiovascular and nervous system. Since the energy requirements of the CNS and peripheral nerves are derived solely from the oxidation of glucose, the nervous system is the first to suffer in thiamine deficiency. Loss of appetite, growth failure, weakness and progressive decline in weight are observed early in B_1 deficiency.

In thiamine deficiency, a form of peripheral neuritis is manifested affecting both the sensory and motor nerves. During the early stages, acute pain of nerves (neuralgia) and sudden painful contractions of the calf muscles (cramps) are common; then thigh muscles become weak and 'toe and foot-drop' develops.

Acute beriberi is of two types depending on whether edema is present or not. When carbohydrate metabolism is impaired in neurons "dry beriberi" results. Extreme weakness, weight loss, numbness and paralysis are the primary symptoms. Severe thiamine deficiency impairs carbohydrate metabolism in the heart and blood vessels, causing congestive heart failure ("wet beriberi"). It is associated with "pitting" edema.

Requirement

Daily intake of 1.0–1.5 mg of thiamine for adults is recommended depending upon carbohydrate intake and muscular activity.

RIBOFLAVIN (VITAMIN B₂)

Introduction

Vitamin B_2 is chemically known as riboflavin. Riboflavin contains ribitol (the alcohol corresponding to ribose) attached to a substituted isoalloxazine (flavin) ring. Riboflavin has orange yellow crystals, soluble in water. It gives yellow green fluorescence.

Food Sources

Riboflavin is widely distributed especially in all leafy vegetables and flesh of mammals. Excellent sources are heart, liver, kidney, milk, eggs, green leafy vegetables and yeast (Fig. 4.15). Cereals have low riboflavin

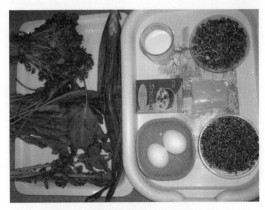
Fig. 4.15: Sources of vitamin B₂

content which increases strikingly on germination.

Functions

Riboflavin forms two coenzymes: FMN-Flavin mononucleotide and FAD-Flavin adenine dinucleotide. FMN and FAD are coenzymes for a class of enzymes called flavin-linked dehydrogenases or flavoproteins which participate in oxidation–reduction reactions concerned with hydrogen and electron transfer.

Deficiency

Riboflavin deficiency signs include cheilosis, glossitis, seborrhic dermatitis and ocular manifestation (corneal vascularization) but mainly mouth, lips and tongue are affected.

Cheilosis: Transverse fissures at the corners of the mouth, raw and scaly lips and finally many vertical deep fissures (Fig. 4.16).

Glossitis: Inflammation of tongue (flattening of papillae), magenta (purple) tongue (Fig. 4.17).

Requirement

The riboflavin requirement is similar to thiamin requirement but depends upon the protein intake.

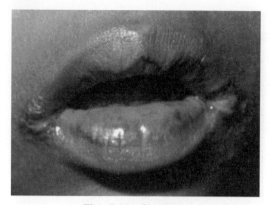

Fig. 4.16: Cheilosis

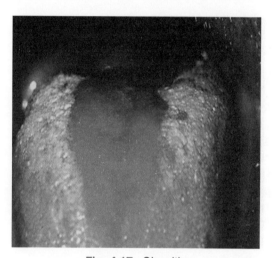

Fig. 4.17: Glossitis

NIACIN (VITAMIN B₃)

Introduction

Niacin is another B complex vitamin known to have coenzyme role. It was called pellagra preventing factor.

Chemically niacin is nicotinic acid. The vitamin activity is also exhibited by its amide, nicotinamide.

Food Sources

Nicotinic acid is present in most foods except in fats and oils. Yeast is the richest source. Other good sources are meat, fish, liver, poultry and grain products, but it is removed during grain processing. Coffee is said to contribute significant amounts of niacin (Fig. 4.18). In some foods, it is present in form that is not absorbable—for example, in corn. It is stable in foods and can survive a reasonable amount of heating, cooking and storage. Amino acid tryptophan of dietary proteins also provides niacin. Animal proteins provide more tryptophan than vegetable proteins (1.4% *versus* 1%).

Functions

Nicotinamide functions as a constituent of two co-enzymes: NAD (Nicotinamide

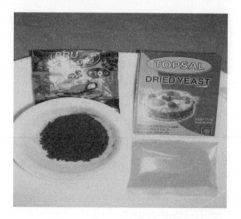

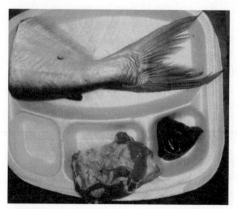

Fig. 4.18: Sources of vitamin B₃ (niacin)

adenine dinucleotide) and NADP (Nicotinamide adenine dinucleotide phosphate).

These coenzymes operate as hydrogen transfer agents in oxidation–reduction reactions by reversible oxidation and reduction of nicotinamide moiety. These coenzymes are part of several enzymes known as pyridine-linked or nicotinamide nucleotide linked dehydrogenases. The NAD linked dehydrogenases are usually associated with aerobic respiratory processes (catabolism) and NADP-linked dehydrogenase with biosynthetic reactions (anabolism).

Deficiency

Niacin deficiency produces pellagra in humans. Pellagra means 'rough skin'. The classical symptoms of pellagra are described as 3Ds: dermatitis, diarrhea and dementia. Dementia is organically caused by impairment of mental functions. The other symptoms are stomatitis and glossitis.

Pellagra is common in areas where maize is the staple diet, because it is low in niacin as well as tryptophan and high in leucine. Sunlight is important precipitating factor in some areas because skin lesions are confined to sun exposed parts of the body, i.e. hands, arms and neck (Fig. 4.19).

Requirement

Niacin requirements are influenced by protein intake as 60 mg of tryptophan is considered to produce 1 mg of niacin. Human requirement is about 20 mg per day.

PYRIDOXAL (VITAMIN B_6)

Introduction

The vitamin B_6 consists of three closely related compounds—pyridoxal, pyridoxine and pyridoxamine which are readily interconvertible biologically and are equally effective. The active form of vitamin B_6 is pyridoxal-5-phosphate, which also occurs in the form, pyridoxamine phosphate. Like niacin, vitamin B_6 contains pyridine ring.

Food Sources

Vitamin B_6 is produced by intestinal microorganisms, but not much of this is absorbed. The vitamin is present in plant and animal tissues. For this reason, dietary deficiency is uncommon. Good sources of vitamin B_6 are yeast, polished rice, wheat, corn and liver (Fig. 4.20). Losses of vitamin B_6 have been observed during heating and storage of some foods. Losses may also occur during processing.

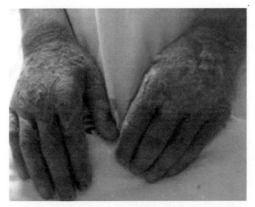

Fig. 4.19: Dermatitis of hands in pellagra

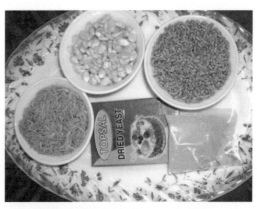

Fig. 4.20: Sources of vitamin B_6

Functions

Pyridoxal is converted into pyridoxal-5-phosphate in the body which serves as coenzyme of several enzymes which are all concerned with amino acid metabolism. The most important of them being decarboxylation and transamination reactions.

1. *Decarboxylation:* Decarboxylation of certain amino acids forms several important compounds in the body, viz. γ-amino butyric acid, 5-hydroxytryptamine or serotonin, histamine and dopamine, etc.

2. *Transamination:* Transamination is transfer or exchange of an alpha-amino group and an alpha-keto group of an α keto acid, thus, producing a new amino acid and new keto acid. It is catalyzed by transaminases, also known as amino transferases, which have pyridoxal phosphate as prosthetic group.

$$R_1-\underset{\underset{NH_2}{|}}{CH}-COOH + R_2-\underset{\underset{O}{\|}}{C}-COOH \rightleftharpoons$$

$$R_1-\underset{\underset{O}{\|}}{C}-COOH + R_2-\underset{\underset{NH_2}{|}}{CH}-COOH$$

Deficiency

Vitamin B_6 is required by all animals. B_6 deficiency results in impaired growth may be due to its wide ranging role in amino acid metabolism. The effect of B_6 deficiency is also noticed on brain metabolism, oxalate metabolism and heme synthesis. Pyridoxal deficiency does not occur normally but can be produced experimentally. Since B_6 coenzymes are involved in many amines which have effect on brain and nerve function, convulsions and peripheral neuropathy was observed in some cases.

B_6 deficiency predisposes to oxalate stone formation in urinary tract of persons. It is explained by increased synthesis of oxalate and hyperoxaluria. Sometimes a hypochromic microcytic anemia is encountered in B_6 deficiency because B_6 coenzymes catalyze reaction leading to heme synthesis.

Requirement

The recommended intake is 2 mg per day. During pregnancy and lactation, 2.5 mg is required.

FOLIC ACID

Introduction

Folic acid was first isolated from spinach leaves. Chemically it is known as pteroyl glutamic acid (PGA) or folacin.

The term folic acid is applied to a number of compounds which contain the following chemical groups: (i) a pteridine nucleus (pyrimidine and pyrazine rings) (ii) p-amino benzoic acid and (iii) L-glutamic acid/acids. It exists in nature as monoglutamate, triglutamate and heptaglutamate which contains one, three and seven glutamic acid molecules, respectively.

Food Sources

Folates are present in a wide variety of plant and animal tissues, but the nutritional availability differs. Rich sources are—yeast, liver, kidney, green leafy vegetables. The food with high availability include bananas, liver and yeast, while food with low availability are orange juice, lettuce, egg yolk, cabbage and soya bean (Fig. 4.21). Like thiamine, this vitamin is labile to cooking. Steaming and frying can result to losses as much as 90%. It is synthesized by intestinal micro-organisms.

Functions

Folic acid coenzymes participate in the synthesis of (a) purine (b) pyrimidine (c) DNA (d) choline and (e) metabolism of some amino acids.

Deficiency

The deficiency of folic acid may arise from dietary inadequacy, malabsorption, antibiotic therapy and increased requirement as

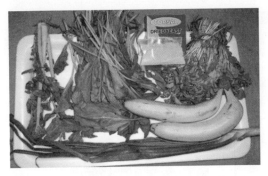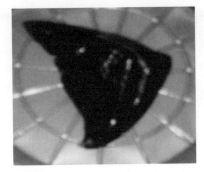

Fig. 4.21: Sources of folic acid

in pregnancy. The participation of folic acid coenzymes in reactions leading to synthesis of choline for phospholipids, amino acids for proteins and purine and pyrimidine for nucleotides, deoxythymidylic acid (dTMP) for DNA, emphasizes its fundamental role in growth and reproduction of cells.

The requirement for this vitamin is generalized throughout the body, but the growth effects are particularly striking in rapidly developing tissues, such as embryonic, hemopoietic and certain types of neoplasms. So in man, folic acid deficiency results in a macrocytic (megaloblastic) anemia which resembles pernicious anemia, except that the nervous involvement of latter condition is absent. Involvement of the gastrointestinal tract may be expressed as diarrhea, glossitis and stomatitis.

Requirement

The recommended daily allowance for adults is 400 µg; this amount is doubled during pregnancy.

CYANOCOBALAMIN—VITAMIN B$_{12}$

Introduction

Vitamin B$_{12}$ or cyanocobalamin was the last B vitamin to be isolated. It was previously named 'extrinsic factor' by Castle as it was required in addition to 'intrinsic factor' to prevent pernicious anemia. Therefore, it was also called anti-pernicious anemia factor.

Vitamin B$_{12}$ was first isolated as cyanocobalamin. It is the only vitamin which contains a metal, that is cobalt.

Food Sources

Vitamin B$_{12}$ is confined to animal food sources. Plants contain no vitamin B$_{12}$. Richest sources are liver and kidney. The vitamin is produced by bacteria and enters human by contaminated foods. Microorganisms in the colon synthesize, but it is not absorbed at that site. The strict vegetarian may develop B$_{12}$ deficiency. The usual dietary sources are meat, fish, eggs and to a lesser extent milk and milk products (Fig. 4.22). Most cooking methods do not destroy B$_{12}$.

Functions

B$_{12}$ coenzymes catalyze mainly two types of reactions. One is in which hydrogen is transferred from one atom to another in the same molecule (intramolecular hydrogen transfer) and the other is intermolecular methyl group transfer in which methyl group of methyl folate is transferred to homocysteine to form methionine.

Deficiency

A deficient intake of vitamin B$_{12}$ occurs in (i) pure vegetarian who refuses to take even

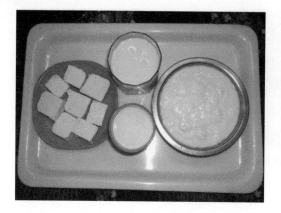 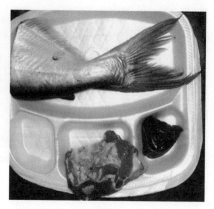

Fig. 4.22: Sources of vitamin B_{12}

milk and milk products (vegans); (ii) in infants when mother breast feed despite deficient intake of animal protein and Vitamin B_{12}. Deficiency of vitamin B_{12} causes pernicious anemia. In man, it is not due to dietary inadequacy of B_{12}, but is due to absence of intrinsic factor in gastric juice (due to atrophy of gastric mucosa) which leads to inadequate intestinal absorption of B_{12}. The ileum is the site of absorption of vitamin B_{12}. Diseases of the ileum, such as regional enteritis, intestinal tuberculosis, celiac syndrome, sprue and resection of distal ileum result in lack of absorption of vitamin B_{12}.

As vitamin B_{12} (and also folic acid) acts to promote development of cells of the erythroid series, beyond the megaloblast stage, its deficiency results in accumulation of megaloblasts in the bone marrow and a macrocytic (megaloblastic) anemia known as pernicious anemia (Fig. 4.23).

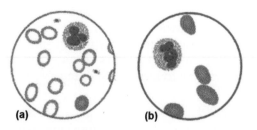

(a)   **(b)**

Fig. 4.23: Blood film of (a) iron deficiency anemia and (b) pernicious anemia (PA)

In addition to anemia, other features are: achlorhydria, achylia gastrica (very little gastric juice), glossitis and degenerative lesions of the posterior and lateral columns of the spinal cord (subacute combined degeneration of the spinal cord) resulting in peripheral sensory disturbances, hyperactive reflexes, ataxia and paralysis. It is inevitably fatal if untreated.

Requirement

The requirement for the normal adult is very small (1 mcg per day) and 1.5 µg / day during pregnancy and lactation.

BIOTIN

Introduction

The existence of vitamin biotin was indicated by the observation that when raw eggs (and not boiled eggs) were fed in large quantities to animals, it caused dermatitis and other symptoms. Raw egg whites contain a protein called avidin, which combines with an essential nutrient and makes it unavailable to the body. Boiling the eggs denatures avidin, rendering it innocuous. This essential nutrient was first called anti-egg white injury factor and later on biotin.

The unique structure of biotin can be divided into two components: (1) a bicyclic ring containing one sulfur and two nitrogen atoms, and (2) a five carbon chain ending in a carboxylate group. Functionally, biotin ring carries an activated CO_2 group and catalyze carboxylation reactions, e.g. acetyl CoA to malonyl CoA and pyruvate to oxaloacetate.

Food Sources

Biotin is widely distributed in food. Excellent sources are egg yolk, kidney, liver, tomatoes, yeast, corn and soya. It is present in free or bound forms. It is liberated from the latter by enzymatic hydrolysis in the gut. The vitamin is heat labile, but much of it is retained in processed foods. Rich sources (600–2000 µg/100 gm) include yeast extracts, liver and other organ meats, soya beans and egg yolk (Fig. 4.24).

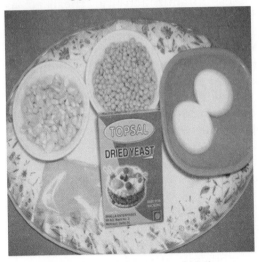

Fig. 4.24: Food sources of biotin

Requirement

The normal requirement of biotin is around 100–200 µg per day which is more than met with ordinary diet.

PANTOTHENIC ACID

Introduction

Pantothenic acid is found everywhere, hence, its deficiency is unknown in man.

Therefore, its vitamin function is of very little importance, however, its role in preventing greying of hairs has been of much interest with the result that hair oils containing it and related compound Panthenol have been in market for a long time.

Food Sources

Pantothenic acid is widely distributed especially in animal tissues. Vegetables and fruits contain less vitamin. Good sources are yeast, polished rice, wheat germ, cereals, legumes and eggs (Fig. 4.25). Intestinal flora also synthesize it.

Requirement

Daily requirement is around 10 mg/day. Some vitamin is lost in heating and processing of food.

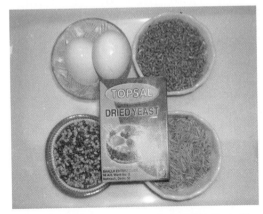

Fig. 4.25: Food sources of pantothenic acid

Functions

Pantothenic acid forms coenzyme, known as coenzyme A, which participates in a number of important reactions in metabolism.

1. Coenzyme A forms acetyl CoA, succinyl CoA and fatty acyl CoA.
2. Coenzyme A participates in oxidative decarboxylation of pyruvate and α-ketoglutarate.

3. Acetyl coenzyme A is used in the synthesis of fatty acids.

4. Acetyl CoA is oxidized in the TCA cycle.

5. Coenzyme A is required for activation of fatty acid for oxidation.

6. Ketone bodies are formed and catabolized through acetyl CoA.

7. Acetyl CoA is used in acetylation reaction, e.g. acetylation of choline to form acetyl choline.

8. Acetyl CoA is starting material for synthesis of cholesterol and from it, other steroid hormones are formed.

9. Coenzyme A forms succinyl CoA which then forms heme.

OTHER VITAMINS

In addition to these compounds, there is no agreement for inclusion of choline, ethanolamine, inositol, para amino benzoic acid and lipoic acid in vitamins. Choline ethanolamine and inositol are lipotropic compounds which prevent accumulation of fat in the liver. p-amino benzoic acid is vitamin for micro-organisms but not man who requires folic acid which contains PABA. Lipoic acid participates in oxidative decarboxylation reactions of pyruvate and α-ketoglutarate in association with thiamine pyrophosphate and others.

VITAMIN ANTAGONISTS

"An anti-vitamin may be defined as any substance that interferes with the synthesis or metabolism of vitamin by a) inactivation or chemical destruction b) irreversible combination c) competitive inhibition."

A number of vitamins are synthesized in intestinal tract such as vitamin K and B complex, thus accounting for at least part of the body requirements. To combat the pathogenic micro-organism growth, chemotherapeutic agents are used in intestinal tract. These agents also destroy bacterial flora and therefore impose a deficiency of the vitamin since they are not being synthesized.

Avidin is a protein occurring in raw egg white which combines with biotin so that it cannot be absorbed. However, a very large intake of raw eggs would be necessary to provide sufficient avidin to provoke biotin deficiency.

Some compounds are closely similar in chemical structure to vitamins but do not possess vitamin activity. These act as vitamin antagonists. They have been used to produce experimental deficiency when the omission of the vitamin from the diet of the experimental subject has not been practical for one reason or another. Only through the use of antagonists, it has been possible to describe symptoms of deficiency of pantothenic acid and vitamin B_6.

Raw fish and bracken fern contain an enzyme, thiaminase, which splits thiamine so that it is rendered ineffective. Thiaminase is inactived by cooking.

Dicoumarin, which has been isolated from sweet clover, acts as vitamin K antagonist and produces hypoprothrombinemia in number of species. It is often used as anti-coagulant.

The summarized information about food sources, biochemical functions and deficiency symptoms of fat soluble vitamin is given in Table 4.1 and of water soluble in Table 4.2.

Table 4.1: Summary of fat soluble vitamins

Vitamins	Food sources	Functions	Deficiency symptoms
Vitamin A	Fish liver oil, green leafy vegetables and carrots for provitamin A	Normal vision	Night blindness, Xerophthalmia, Keratomalacia
Vitamin D	Cod liver oil, other fish liver oils, egg yolk and sunlight	Absorption of Ca, bone formation, regulation of Ca and P in bones and kidney	Rickets (impaired mineralization of bones), osteomalacia (demineralization of bones)
Vitamin E	Wheat germ oil, egg, meat, fish, corn oil, soybean oil	Anti-oxidants, anti-sterility	Human deficiency in animals rare
Vitamin K	Green leafy vegetables, tomatoes, cheese, fish, egg yolk	Prothrombin synthesis	Impaired blood clotting, uncontrolled hemorrhage

Table 4.2: Summary of water soluble vitamins

Vitamins	Food sources	Functions	Deficiency symptoms
Vitamin B complex			
Thiamine	Unrefined cereal grain,	Aldehyde group removal or transfer	Beriberi (peripheral neuropathy), congestive heart failure
Riboflavin	Milk, eggs, green leafy vegetables, beans, nuts and meat	Hydrogen transfer	Chielosis, glossitis
Niacin	Meat, chicken, coffee	Hydrogen transfer	Pellagra (dermatitis diarrhea, dementia)
Pyridoxine	Unpolished rice, wheat, corn	Amino group transfer	Impaired brain metabolism, hyperoxaluria, anemia, peripheral neuropathy
Biotin	Egg yolk, tomatoes, corn, soya	Carboxyl group removal or transfer	Dermatitis
Pantothenic acid	Unpolished rice, wheat, cereals, legumes, eggs	Acyl group transfer	Deficiency not reported
Folic acid	Green leafy vegetables, specially spinach	One C unit transfer	Megaloblastic anemia
Cabalamin	Animal food sources	1, 2 hydrogen shift, methyl group carrier	Pernicious anemia
Vitamin C	Amla, citrus fruits	Coenzyme in hydroxylation of proline in collagen synthesis, anti-oxidant	Poor wound healing, loosening of teeth, bleeding gums, anemia

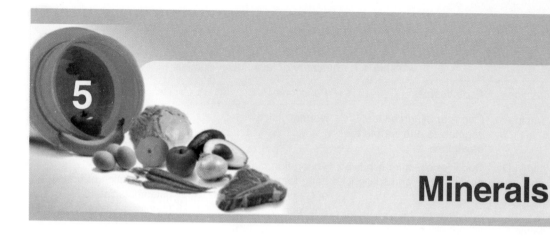

Minerals

INTRODUCTION

The amount of inorganic matter in human body is less than 5%. The study of these compounds is the subject matter of this chapter. This constitutes what some people prefer to call 'Inorganic Biochemistry'. Although present in much smaller quantity, minerals play very important role in the body.

There are numbers of inorganic minerals present in the body. The following is a list of essential elements:

Sodium (Na), potassium (K), calcium (Ca), magnesium (Mg), phosphorous (P), sulphur (S), iron (Fe), iodine (I), manganese (Mn), molybdenum (Mo), zinc (Zn), fluorine (F), chromium (Cr), nickel (Ni), silicon (Si), strontium (Sn), selenium (Se) and vanadium (V).

Their amount in the body varies considerably from kilogram (calcium) to gram (chloride) to milligram (copper) and even microgram (cobalt) or even less (chromium).

The inorganic elements have various functions in the body as shown in Table 5.1.

MACROELEMENTS

These minerals are required in comparatively larger amounts in the diet, generally greater than 100 mg/day. There are seven essential principal elements–calcium, magnesium, sodium, potassium, phosphorous, sulphur and chlorine.

Sodium

About 100 g of sodium is present in the body. About one-third is in the skeleton as fixed salts. It is the major cation of extra cellular fluid (average volume is 14 liters in adults). Average level of sodium in plasma is about 330 mg/100 ml (143 mmol/L).

Table 5.1: Functions of inorganic elements

Functions	Minerals
1. Structural	Calcium, magnesium, phosphorous
2. Membrane	Sodium, potassium (principal cation of extracellular fluids and intracellular fluids, respectively)
3. Function as prosthetic groups in enzymes	Cobalt, copper, iron, molybdenum, selenium, zinc
4. Regulatory role or role in hormone action	Calcium, iodine, magnesium, manganese, sodium, potassium

Sources

Sodium is contributed mainly by common salt. Cheese, fish and shell fish as well as meat and eggs are good sources of sodium (Fig. 5.1).

Cereals, fruits and vegetables are low in salt. However, the amount of salt added in processing or fermentation of food can be considerable.

Sodium has several functions in the body, for example:

1. Regulation of acid–base balance in association with chloride and bicarbonate.
2. Maintenance of osmotic pressure of body fluids thus preserving excessive fluid loss.
3. Preservation of normal irritability of muscles together with other ions.
4. Preservation of normal permeability of the cells.

The main source of sodium in diet is common salt used in cooking and seasoning. Ingested foods contain additional sodium. Sodium is readily absorbed so that feces contain very little except in diarrhea. Sodium is consumed in much larger amounts than required, so the excess is excreted in urine.

There is evidence to link dietary intake of sodium with development of high blood pressure, but not all individuals are susceptible. In such patients, moderate sodium restriction may be helpful in lowering blood pressure. About 5 gm NaCl per day is recommended for adults without history of hypertension and 1g NaCl per day with family history of hypertension.

The metabolism of sodium is influenced by the adrenocortical steroids. Aldosterone increases the reabsorption of sodium (and chloride) by the renal tubules and decreases their excretion by other routes. Therefore, in adrenocortical insufficiency (Addison's disease—Fig. 5.2), a decrease of serum sodium (hyponatremia) occurs.

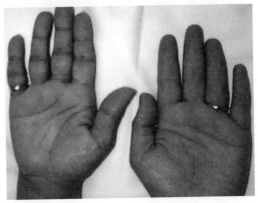

Fig. 5.2: Addison's disease—patients have darkening (hyperpigmentation) of the skin

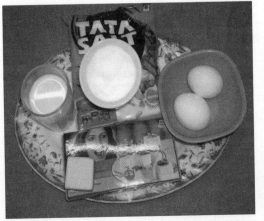 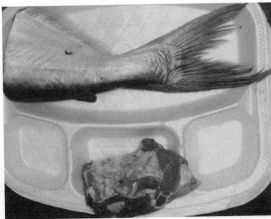

Fig. 5.1: Food sources of sodium

This is also found in chronic renal disease due to poor tubular reabsorption and excessive diarrhea. Severe hyponatremia may cause the symptoms such as dehydration; fall in blood volume and blood pressure and finally circulatory failure.

Hypernatremia or increase in serum sodium occurs in hyperactivity of adrenal cortex (Cushing's disease or syndrome). Its symptoms are increased retention of water in the body called oedema (Fig. 5.3), increase in blood volume and blood pressure.

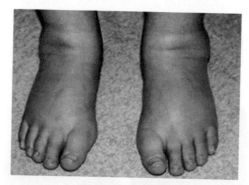

Fig. 5.3: Oedema

Unless the individual is well adopted to a high environmental temperature, extreme sweating may cause the heat stroke due to considerable loss of sodium. The symptoms are headache, nausea, diarrhea, muscular cramps of the extremities and abdomen.

Potassium

About 250 g of potassium is present in the adult human body. About 90% is in the cells and the remainder in the extracellular fluids. Thus, potassium is the principal cation of the intracellular fluid (volume about 35 liters). For example, plasma contains 20 mg%, whole blood 200 mg%, muscles 250 to 400 mg% and nerves 530 mg%.

The functions of potassium in the body are (1) within the cells, potassium functions for acid–base balance, osmotic pressure and water retention and (2) in extracellular fluid, it influences muscle activity, notably cardiac muscles.

Potassium is widely distributed in the food, hence, dietary deficiency is unlikely to occur. Average intake varies from 2 to 4 gm per day.

Kidney is the principal organ of excretion. Potassium is filtered in the glomeruli and also secreted by the tubules.

The variations of potassium level in extracellular fluid occur by muscle and glycogen synthesis and breakdown. These variations in extracellular fluid potassium influence the activity of the cardiac and striated muscles.

Sources

Meat is a source of potassium. Milk, vegetables and fruits are good sources. For example, green leafy vegetables, tomatoes, amla, sweet lime, lemon, fennel, turnip greens, mushrooms, carrots, green beans, banana and papaya are notable sources (Fig. 5.4).

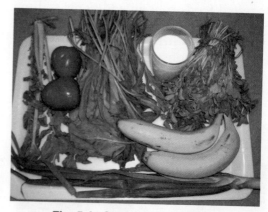

Fig. 5.4: Sources of potassium

Hyperkalemia (high serum potassium): It is caused by Addison's disease, renal failure, advanced dehydration and shock. The symptoms are cardiac and central nervous system depression. Cardiac symptoms are bradycardia and cardiac arrest. CNS symptoms are mental confusion, weakness, numbness, etc.

Hypokalemia (low serum potassium): It is caused by malnutrition, gastrointestinal losses, metabolic alkalosis and Cushing's syndrome. The symptoms of hypokalemia are muscle weakness, irritability, paralysis, tachycardia and dilation of the heart.

Chlorine (as Chloride)

Chloride occurs intra and extracellularly. Plasma contains, on an average, 365 mg/100 ml (103 mmols/L) and cells contain 190 mg/100 ml (53 mmols/L).

As a part of sodium chloride, chloride is essential for (1) water balance, (2) osmotic pressure regulation, and (3) acid–base equilibrium. Independent of NaCl, chloride forms HCl in the stomach.

In the diet, chloride occurs as NaCl, therefore, intake of chloride would be adequate as long as sodium intake is adequate. The intake, output and metabolism of both are inseparable.

Abnormalities of sodium metabolism are generally accompanied by abnormalities in chloride metabolism. When losses of sodium are excessive, as in diarrhea, profuse sweating, certain endocrine disturbances (Addison's disease) and chloride deficiency is also observed.

In vomiting, loss of gastric HCl occurs, leading to loss of chloride in excess of sodium.

As sodium contributes the largest fraction of the total cation of the extracellular fluids (142/155) and chloride constitutes the largest fraction of total anions of the plasma (103/155), the maintenance of normal pH depends largely upon the presence of normal concentrations of sodium and chloride.

The importance of a proper balance between Na, K, Mg and Ca in the maintenance of normal neuromuscular irritability and excitability is well known.

Calcium

Adult human body contains about 1.5 kg of calcium, which is the largest amount for any cation. 99% of this calcium is present in bones and teeth and the remaining is in the body fluids.

Apart from bone formation, ionic calcium is of great importance in blood coagulation, in the functions of heart, muscles and nerves, in the permeability of membranes and for the activity of certain enzymes.

Sources

In general, calcium is found primarily in dairy products, meat and certain fish. Milk and cheese are the most important dietary sources of calcium, because calcium-phosphorous ratio is optimal for absorption of this element. Other good sources are egg yolk, lentils, beans, nuts, cabbage and cauliflower (Fig. 5.5).

In animal products, calcium is largely bound to protein whereas in vegetables, it is complexed with organic anions, such as phytates and oxalates. The protein in animal food must be digested for calcium absorption to occur. On the other hand, the organic anions in vegetables are not digested and poorly absorbed. Thus, vegetable calcium is less available than that from animal sources.

Absorption

Calcium is absorbed in the intestine under the influence of Vitamin D. The active form

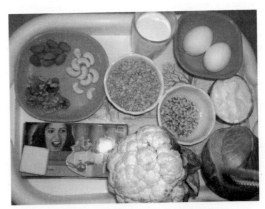

Fig. 5.5: Food sources of calcium

of vitamin D-1, 25-dihydroxycholecalciferol (calcitriol) is taken up by the intestinal mucosal cells, where it stimulates the production of specific mRNA, which is concerned with the production of calcium binding proteins. The other factors which affect calcium absorption are discussed below. Many of these are common to absorption of another divalent cation, ferrous iron.

1. *pH:* Calcium is well absorbed at the normal pH of the intestinal contents. If the pH becomes more alkaline, calcium absorption is suppressed.

2. *Phosphate:* Excess of phosphate lowers calcium absorption by forming insoluble calcium phosphate.

3. *Phytic acid:* Phytic acid present in cereals interferes with the absorption of calcium by forming insoluble salt.

4. *Oxalates:* Oxalic acid and oxalates present in several foods lower calcium absorption by precipitating calcium as insoluble calcium oxalate.

5. *Vitamin D:* Vitamin D promotes absorption of calcium from the intestine by stimulating *de novo* synthesis of calcium binding proteins.

6. *Fatty acids:* Impaired fat absorption produces much free fatty acids in the intestine, which lowers calcium absorption by forming insoluble calcium soaps.

Metabolism

There is virtually no calcium in red blood cells, all is present in plasma. Normal level of total calcium is 9–11.5 mg/100 ml. Calcium exists in plasma in two fractions.

a. Diffusible (50–60% of total) which includes ionized calcium and calcium complexed with citrate and phosphate.

b. Non-diffusible (40–50%) or protein bound. Plasma calcium is mainly used for the formation of bone salts. Bone is not static deposit of calcium and phosphorous. These ions from plasma exchange with

those on the surface of bones, and complete exchange of plasma calcium occurs within 2–3 minutes.

Calcium is reabsorbed in the tubules so only small amount is excreted in urine (200 mg). Unabsorbed calcium is passed in feces. Parathyroid hormone (PTH) increases serum calcium while calcitonin (CT) hormone of thyroid decreases it. The main features of regulation of blood calcium are shown in Fig. 5.6.

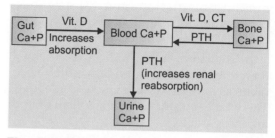

Fig. 5.6: Regulation of blood calcium and phosphorous

Variation of Blood Calcium in Health and Disease

Normal level of calcium in plasma or serum is about 9–11.5 mg% (4.5–5.8 mEq/liter). Plasma inorganic phosphorous level in children is about 4–6 mg% (2.4–3.6 mEq/liter) and in adults 3–4.5 mg% (1.8–2.6 mEq/liter). The Ca × P product is important in ossification. The Ca × P product is over 50 in normal children and about 30 to 40 in normal adults. This product is very much reduced in rickets and osteomalacia.

A decrease in the ionized fraction (5.4–6.6 mg%) of serum calcium due to any reason causes tetany. This may be due to an increase in the pH of blood or to a lack of calcium because of poor absorption from intestine, decreased dietary intake, increased renal excretion or parathyroid deficiency. Increased retention of phosphorous, as in renal tubular disease, also predisposes to low serum calcium. Other disease conditions associated with hypercalcemia and hypo-calcemia are discussed below.

Hypercalcemia

It results in:

1. *Hyperparathyroidism:* Serum calcium varies between 12 and 22 mg%.
2. *Multiple Myeloma:* Serum calcium varies from normal to 20 mg% due to destruction of bone with liberation of its minerals.
3. *Cancer:* Serum calcium is usually normal but values as high as 22 mg% may be obtained in cases of extensive osteolytic metastatic involvement of the skeleton.

Hypocalcemia

It results in:

1. *Hypoparathyroidism:* Serum calcium is decreased in hypoparathyroidism.
2. *Tetany:* Decrease in serum ionized calcium due to any reason give rise to tetany. Total serum calcium is usually between 7 and 8 mg% in latent and 4–6 mg% in manifest tetany.
3. *Rickets and osteomalacia:* In early cases, serum calcium is normal, then it falls. If calcium intake is low, hypocalcemia occurs which give rise to tetany (Fig. 5.7).
4. *Steatorrhoea:* Defective absorption of fat, fatty acids and vitamin D is the cause of hypocalcemia of steatorrhoea.

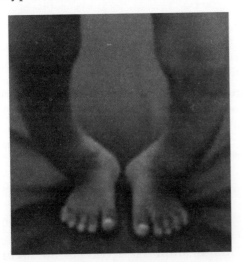

Fig. 5.7: Rickets

5. *Nephrotic syndrome:* Serum calcium may be low due to loss of non-diffusible, protein bound calcium in urine.
6. *Chronic renal failure:* Fall in serum calcium (4–6 mg%) is due to retention of phosphate (12–20 mg%) by kidney. Tetany may also occur.
7. *Pregnancy:* Serum calcium may fall during late pregnancy or lactation owing to increased demand of calcium, phosphorous and vitamin D.

Requirement: The suggested requirement is shown in Table 5.2.

Table 5.2: Recommended dietary allowance for calcium	
Age group	mg/day
Infants (0 to 12 months)	500–600
Children (1 to 9 yrs)	400–500
Children (10 to 15 yrs)	600–700
Children (16 to 19 yrs)	500–600
Adults	400–500
Pregnancy and lactation	1000

Phosphorous

Distribution

Adults contain about 400–700 g of phosphorous, 80% of which is combined with calcium in bones and teeth. The rest is in combination with other elements in other tissues.

Sources

Phosphorous is a constituent of all cells and is thus present in all foods. Both organic and inorganic forms of phosphorous are handled alike, due to the presence of alkaline phosphate in the intestinal tract. Milk is an excellent source of both calcium and phosphorous with a ratio about 1:1. Human milk is relatively low in phosphorous while cow's milk has 5–6 times to it. Other important sources are eggs, meat and fish (Fig. 5.8). Vegetables are fair sources. Cereals, pulses and nuts are poor sources as the large part exists in the form of phytic acid. Generally, the distribution of phosphorous and calcium in food is similar.

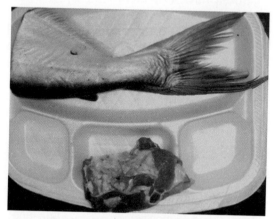

Fig. 5.8: Sources of phosphorous

Functions

Important functions of phosphorous are:
1. It functions in formation of bones and teeth.
2. It forms high energy phosphate compounds, e.g. creatine phosphate.
3. It forms nucleoproteins which are present in every cell.
4. It participates in cell structure as phospholipids.
5. It influences acid base balance as Na_2HPO_4 and NaH_2PO_4.

Metabolism

Ordinary diet contains phosphorous from 1.5 to 3 times to calcium; while the optimal ratio for children is 1:1 and for adults 1:2 (as Ca: P). Absorption occurs in small intestine as inorganic phosphate. Retention is about 10–40%, depending on calcium and vitamin D. Serum inorganic phosphorous level in children is 4–6 mg% and 3–4.5 mg% in adults. Parathormone inhibits renal tubular reabsorption of inorganic phosphate resulting into a lowered plasma level.

Hyperphosphatemia has been observed in hypoparathyroidism due to excessive tubular reabsorption of phosphate and in renal failure due to renal functional insufficiency in which case values as high as 40 mg% may be observed. Hypophosphatemia is found in rickets, osteomalacia, vitamin D resistant rickets, hyperparathyroidism and Fanconi's Syndrome.

Requirement

The recommended requirement of phosphorous is roughly equal to or 1.5 times that of calcium. The RDA of 500 mg for children and 800–1200 mg for adults is recommended. There is no risk of phosphorous shortage in a normal diet, unless large amounts of white flour are consumed as the main cereal.

Magnesium

Occurrence of magnesium is widespread in both plant and animal tissues. The total body concentration of magnesium in a healthy adult is about 20–28 g. More than half (53%) of the body magnesium is in bone as magnesium phosphate $Mg_3 (PO_4)_2$ and almost all the rest in soft tissue.

Sources

Magnesium is highly concentrated in all cells and thus present in most foods. Magnesium is bound by protein and phosphate. In chlorophyll of green plants and vegetables, it is complexed with porphyrin. Hard water contain substantial amount. Foods rich in magnesium include meat, seafood, green vegetables, dairy products, nuts and cereals (Fig. 5.9).

Functions

1. Being part of the bone tissue, magnesium has an important structural function.
2. Magnesium is involved in several essential metabolic reactions.

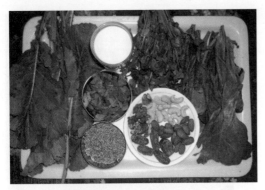

Fig. 5.9: Sources of magnesium

a. Mg^{2+} binds to substrate, thereby forming a complex with which the enzyme interacts as in the reaction of the kinase enzymes with Mg ATP.

b. The magnesium plays an important role in glycolysis, the citric acid cycle, gluconeogenesis, lipid metabolism, amino acid metabolism and nucleic acid metabolism.

c. Magnesium is important in energy metabolism since ATP. The free energy currency for all the cellular processes exists in all cells primarily as MgATP.

Requirement

Since absorption of magnesium is very low (about 30–40%), daily requirement should allow for individual variation: 350 mg/day for male and 280 mg/day in adult female is recommended in USA.

MICROELEMENTS

Microelements occur in living tissues in minute amounts. Other popular names used include 'minor minerals' or 'oligo-elements' (from the Greek 'oligos' meaning scanty). The microminerals are required in less than 100 mg/day.

The microelements may be sub-divided into three groups:

1. Essential trace elements: iron, copper, iodine, zinc, manganese, cobalt, fluorine, molybdenum, selenium and chromium. These have been shown to be dietary essential vital to the enzymic processes of the living cell.

2. Possibly essential trace elements: nickel, tin, vanadium, cadmium, silicon, barium, strontium. They exhibit some metabolic activity, revealed by both in vivo and in vitro studies.

3. Non-essential trace elements: aluminium, boron, lead, mercury, fluorine and arsenic.

Iron

Iron is an essential element. Its deficiency in man causes iron deficiency anemia which is very common disease. The metabolism of iron is unique in the respect that it has a closed system in the body, that is, its content in the body is regulated by absorption rather than excretion, unlike other minerals.

Although present in minute amounts, iron plays very important role. Its function is mainly concerned with respiration, i.e. transport and delivery of oxygen by hemoglobin, and hydrogen and electron transport in ETC by cytochromes. Both are iron-porphyrin protein.

Total body iron content is about 4–6 gm, more than 50% of which is present as heme in hemoglobin, myoglobin in muscles, cytochromes and the enzymes-catalase and peroxidase. The remaining iron is present as non-heme compounds which are usually protein-bound. The important ones are ferritin and hemosiderin for storage of iron and transferrin present for transport of iron.

Iron occurs in food as heme as well as non-heme form. The former is found in animal food and the latter in the plant food.

Sources

The important animal food sources are liver, spleen, muscles, egg yolk, bone marrow and fish as these contain heme iron which is well

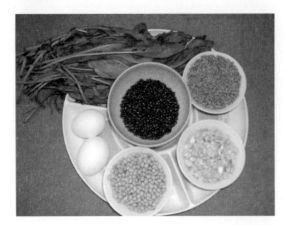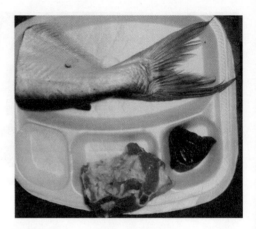

Fig. 5.10: Food sources of iron

absorbed. In vegetarian food, iron is richly present in whole wheat, corn, black gram, soya bean, spinach and other green leafy vegetables, wherein present in ferric salts or ferric organic compounds, which is not well absorbed (Fig. 5.10).

Absorption and Transport

The absorption of iron actually takes place in duodenum or proximal jejunum.

The animal food contains mainly heme iron. Heme is believed to be transported into enterocyte by heme transporter. In the intestinal mucosal cell, iron is released from heme by heme oxidase.

Food especially of plant origin contains mainly inorganic iron salts or non-heme iron. By HCl of stomach, non-heme food iron is released in the form of ferric ion or loosely bound iron. Peptic digestion of proteins is believed to aid in it. HCl is necessary to keep the iron salts in solution. Only ferrous iron is absorbed so reducing substances of food, like, ascorbic acid and cysteine promote iron absorption. On the other hand, phytic acid, oxalates and phosphates present in food inhibit absorption of iron by forming unabsorbable complexes with them.

The released ferrous iron is then transported into the enterocyte by the specific iron transporter. Some of the intracellular ferrous iron is converted into ferric iron and bound to ferritin. The rest of the iron binds to the ferrous transporter and transported to the interstitial fluid. In the plasma, ferrous iron is converted to ferric iron by ceruloplasmin and incorporated into iron transport protein, transferrin. This protein has a very high affinity for iron and binds two atoms of iron per molecule. This is taken up by reticulocytes in bone marrow for hemoglobin synthesis or reticuloendothelial cells in liver, bone marrow, spleen, etc. for storage.

Normal healthy persons have about 75–150 ug Fe/100 ml of plasma. However, the total iron binding capacity of plasma is much more, around 250–400 ug Fe/100 ml. The difference between these values represents unsaturated iron binding capacity of plasma. Thus, normally only 30–40% of plasma transferrin has bound iron. This fraction is called saturation percentage.

Storage, Metabolism and Excretion

Iron is stored in the RE cells of liver (around 700 mg), spleen and bone marrow in the form of a water soluble protein ferritin. When iron content of ferritin is increased, it is converted into hemosiderin. Ferritin and hemosiderin are not static deposits of iron but are in dynamic equilibrium. Hemoglobin regeneration occurs upon blood loss by mobilisation of these stores.

The sum total of iron metabolism is shown in the diagram (Fig. 5.11). About 27 mg of iron is turned over every day. Of this, about 20 mg is obtained from breakdown of red blood cells, 1–2 mg from newly absorbed iron and remainder from the iron stores. Iron is utilized for hemoglobin synthesis by bone marrow, additional amount is stored in tissue and very little is excreted out of body.

There is very little excretion of iron except in cases of losses of blood due to physiological or pathological causes. As iron is bound to protein in plasma (transferrin), it is not lost in urine (less than 0.4 mg/day). Dermal losses are negligible. Unabsorbed iron is passed in the stool.

Iron is mainly lost from the body when there is blood loss in any form. This may be physiological as in case of menstruation or pregnancy or pathological as in hemorrhages or intestinal worms. Theoretically, on an average, females lose about 0.5–1.0 mg Fe/day on account of menstruation. Similarly, it is concluded that each pregnancy entails a net loss of 500 mg iron. Although milk is poor in iron, lactation for 6 months accounts for loss of approximately 180 mg of iron from the lactating mother.

Functions

1. The major function of iron is formation of hemoglobin. In respiration process, when oxygen enters the lungs, it combines with the iron containing protein, hemoglobin, present in RBCs forming the complex oxyhemoglobin. On reaching the tissues, the complex dissociates releasing oxygen. Simultaneously, CO_2 formed as a waste product in catabolic reaction in the tissues, enters RBC and combine with hemoglobin to form hemoglobin carbamate. On reaching lungs, hemoglobin carbamate dissociates, releasing CO_2, which is exhaled.

2. In muscles, oxygen is combined with iron containing muscles protein, myoglobin. When strenuous exercise markedly lowers the oxygen content of muscle cells, myoglobin releases oxygen for mitochondrial synthesis of ATP, permitting continued muscular activity.

3. Iron is a part of heme, a constituent of enzyme peroxidase and catalase which catalyzes oxidation and reduction reaction. Physiologically, these two enzymes are very important since they bring about degradation of toxic peroxide molecules as

$$H_2O_2 + AH_2 \longrightarrow 2H_2O + A$$
$$2H_2O_2 \longrightarrow 2H_2O + O_2$$

Accumulation of peroxide can lead to generation of free radicals (ROO^*, RO^*, OH^*), which in turn can disrupt membrane and could cause cancer and atherosclerosis.

4. Iron, as a part of heme, is present in various cytochromes. Cytochrome is component of the mitochondrial electron transport chain. Here they function as carrier of electron from flavoprotein on the one hand to cytochrome oxidase on the other. In liver microsome, cytochrome P_{450} and b_5 play an important role in detoxification (converting toxic compounds to non-toxic intermediates).

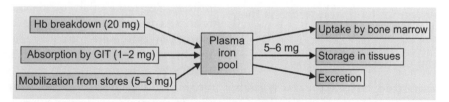

Fig. 5.11: Overview of iron metabolism

Pathology

Deficiency: The deficiency of iron causes iron deficiency anemia which is of hypochromic microcytic type due to decreased heme synthesis. The children and women, especially in reproductive age, are at greater risk. The most frequent causes of iron deficiency are inadequate intake, malabsorption or blood loss in some form. In children, intestinal worms are the main cause of blood loss. In women, it is menstrual bleeding, repeated pregnancy and childbirth and sometimes prolonged lactation.

Iron deficiency is a concern because:

- Iron deficiency can delay normal infant motor function (normal activity and movement) or mental function (normal thinking and processing skills).
- Iron deficiency anemia during pregnancy can increase risk for small or early (preterm) babies. Small or early babies are more likely to have health problems or die in the first year of life than infants who are born full term and are not small.
- Iron deficiency can cause fatigue that impairs the ability to do physical work in adults. Iron deficiency may also affect memory or other mental function in teens.

Excess: As iron has a closed system in the body, iron overload can occur by repeated mismatched blood transfusions or hemolytic anemia. Iron overload also occurs in a genetic disease hemochromatosis.

Hemochromatosis

It is a genetic disease in which the affected person has inherited ability to absorb much greater per cent of food iron which is then deposited in the skin, pancreas and liver giving rise to bronzed coloration, diabetes mellitus and cirrhosis, respectively.

Recommended dietary allowance: Recommended dietary iron intake for Indians by ICMR (1981) is given in Table 5.3.

Table 5.3: Recommended iron intake for Indians ICMR (1981)

	Iron (MG)
Men	24
Women	32
Pregnancy	40
Lactation	32
Infants	1 mg/kg
Children	20–35

Iodine

Iodine is an important essential element. Insufficient quantity of iodine in the diet results in the diseases *Goiter* as shown in Fig. 5.12a. Goiter is characterized by enlarged thyroid glands, which becomes visible in the region of the neck. It occurs when soil and water have low levels of iodine and consequently the food (plants and animals sources) and water we consume are not able to meet our daily requirements. This is also associated with *Cretinism*. Cretinism as shown in Fig. 5.12b is a condition originating in fetal life or early infancy due to severe thyroid deficiency, characterized by stunting of physical growth and decreased mental development. Since iodine is a micronutrient, the very small amount required can easily be met by using iodized salt.

Sources

Iodine is present in the food in the form of iodides. Sea food—fish, oysters, crabs and even sea plants are rich sources. Other sources of iodine are iodized table salt and drinking water. Normal daily intake of iodine is about 100–200 mg, same as recommended dietary allowances. Goitrogens in the diet (e.g. fluorides) will decrease iodine uptake by thyroid glands.

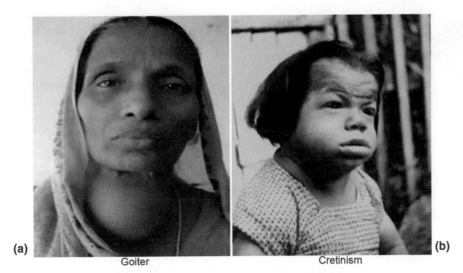

(a)   (b)
Goiter   Cretinism

Fig. 5.12a and b: Iodine deficiency disorders

Functions

The only known function of iodine in the body is formation of thyroid hormones—thyroxine-tetraiodothyroxine (T_4) and triiodothyroxine (T_3). So, iodine metabolism and thyroid function are closely associated. The role of thyroid hormones includes:

1. *Thermogenesis and oxygen consumption:* Increased heat production and oxygen consumption are characteristics of most tissues responding to thyroid hormones (brain, testes and spleen excluded). Thus, thyroid hormone activity is intimately related to metabolic rate (BMR).

2. *Metabolic effects of T_3 and T_4:* Thyroid hormone effects on carbohydrate metabolism involve increased intestinal absorption of glucose balanced by increased glucose utilization. It also alters the metabolism of proteins, lipids, electrolyte and water.

Deficiency

Inadequate supply of iodine in the diet causes goiter, which is actually the enlargement of the thyroid glands in an attempt to trap and utilize more of the Iodine. Goiter may be either a simple enlargement of the gland without hyperactivity (simple goiter) (Fig.5.12a) or enlargement of gland with hyperthyroidism (toxic goiter). Simple goiter is common where the soil and water are low in iodine. The treatment with iodine or sodium iodide is effective. Goiter is very common in many countries all over the world including India—West Bengal, Maharashtra, Rajasthan, Kerala and Karnataka. About million people are actually suffering from deficiency in India.

Copper

The healthy human adult body has about 50–120 mg of total copper, located mostly in bone, liver, kidney and muscles. Copper present in plasma is transported bound to a protein called ceruloplasmin.

Sources

The richest sources are shell fish, oysters and crabs. Next most abundant sources are nuts and legumes, dried fruits and cocoa. Poor sources include dairy products, sugar and honey (Fig. 5.13). The usual vegetarian diet contains 24 mg/day.

The absorption of copper is less than 10%. However, daily need of 2–3 mg is obtained from an average diet. It is transported to liver bound to plasma albumin where it is

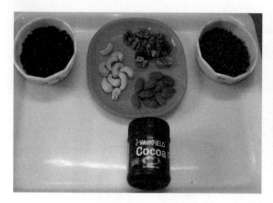
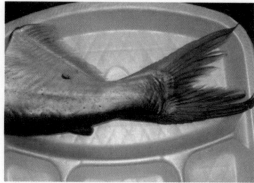

Fig. 5.13: Food sources of copper

incorporated into a specific copper-binding protein ceruloplasmin. This protein exports copper to other tissues.

Copper is the constituent of several enzymes (oxidases) and proteins, e.g. ferroxidase I (ceruloplasmin), erythro-cuprin found in RBCs, cerebrocuprin (found in brain), cytochrome oxidase, monoamine oxidase, lysyl oxidase, superoxide dismutase, etc. Plasma ceruloplasmin has ferroxidase activity, so it oxidizes ferrous ion into ferric ion for incorporation into iron–transport protein transferrin. The enzyme xylyl oxidase is responsible for forming cross links between collagen/elastin fibers.

Copper deficiency is uncommon but whenever occur naturally or experimentally develop hypochromic microcytic anemia due to its role in iron storage, transport and mobilization from stores.

An inherited disease of copper metabolism is Wilson's disease. It is characterized by excessive absorption of copper leading to its deposition in liver, kidney and brain causing liver cirrhosis, kidney damage and neurologic disturbances, respectively.

Zinc

Zinc is an essential element although human body contains only 2 g. Dietary absorption is only 5–10% due to interfering ions—phosphate, phytate and calcium.

Sources

The richest sources are oysters, crabs and shell fish. Zinc content of food varies with the soil and fertilizers in which the foods are grown (Fig. 5.14). In general, the zinc is proportionate to protein intake, since muscles meat and sea birds have the highest content. The vegetable sources contain zinc but due to anions, they are not absorbed.

The amount of zinc in daily diet is around 6–12 mg/dl which is adequate to meet the requirement.

Zinc is a constituent of many metallo-enzymes whose activity is reduced in zinc deficiency. Important ones are alcohol

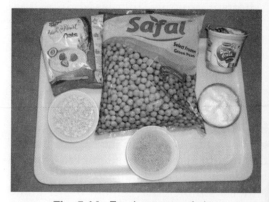

Fig. 5.14: Food sources of zinc

dehydrogenase, alkaline phosphatase, DNA polymerase and RNA polymerase. Thus, zinc has an important role in nucleic acid metabolism and growth failure and poor wound healing is seen in zinc deficiency. Because of it being part of alkaline phosphatase, zinc deficiency causes weak bone formation and skeleton development.

Zinc deficiency has been reported to cause growth failure (dwarfism) and hypogonadism (retarded gonadal development) in Egypt and Iran in adolescent boys. Zinc deficiency is believed to be associated with poor wound healing.

Good sources include asparagus, lamb, beef, green peas, yogurt, oats, pumpkin seeds, sesame seeds (Fig. 5.14).

Fluorine

Like other ionic trace elements (sodium, selenium), the sources of food (where it is grown) is more important than the type of food, as regards fluoride. Sea food is especially rich in it. Tea is the other food naturally high in fluoride. Water is also the major sources of fluoride. Surface water contains 1 ppm or less, deep water contains 4–8 ppm (Fig. 5.15).

Fluorine, as fluoride, has been considered essential, because of its well known effects on prevention of dental caries and in maintenance of normal skeleton. At an optimum level of 1–2 ppm, it causes mottling of enamel of teeth and prevents decay (Fig. 5.16). It is deposited in bones as calcium fluorapatite. Schwarz found fluoride to be essential for growth and development. The concentration of fluorine in plasma is homeostatically controlled at 0.1–0.2 ppm. Daily intake of fluoride is about 4–5 mg.

Fluorosis is toxic manifestation of excess fluoride in drinking water and is a serious public health problem. It is quite prevalent in India, China, Argentina and Africa. It is estimated that approximately 20–25 million

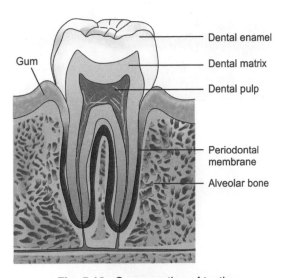

Fig. 5.16: Cross-section of teeth

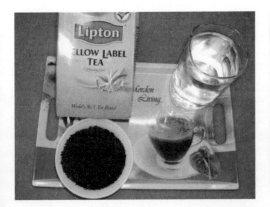
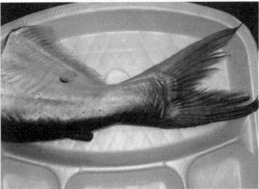

Fig. 5.15: Food sources of fluorine

people suffer from fluorosis in 13 states of India including Rajasthan and Delhi. If the drinking water contains 3–5 ppm fluoride, it causes dental fluorosis, which is characterized by discolored teeth (Fig. 5.17). Excessive amount of fluoride (> 10 ppm) in drinking water causes skeletal fluorosis (Fig. 5.18). "Knock knee" and "bow legs" occur which cripples the person. The treatment of water with lime and alum is recommended to remove excess fluoride from it.

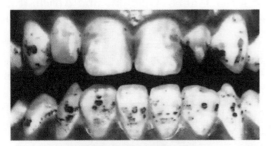

Fig. 5.17: Dental fluorosis

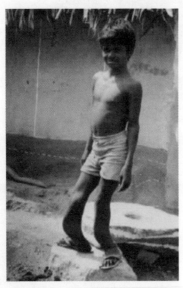

Fig. 5.18: Skeletal fluorosis

Chromium

All plant and animal tissues contain chromium. Dietary chromium occurs in multiple valence states. Most of the chromium in the food is in trivalent state (Cr^{3+}). Hexavalent element of chromium is poorly absorbed in the intestine. Chromium is a bone seeking element and its uptake in bone appears to be rapid. Besides bone, chromium accumulates in spleen, kidney and liver.

Sources

Brewer's yeast is the richest source. Other sources are meat products, dairy products and eggs (Fig. 5.19). Leafy vegetables contain chromium in unabsorbable form. Rice and sugar are poor sources. The safe intake is 50–200 mg.

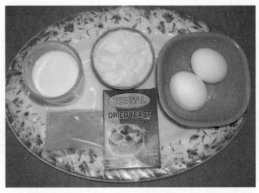

Fig. 5.19: Food sources of chromium

Chromium is now considered an essential element. It was demonstrated that trivalent chromium in the liver is converted into organic compound, named glucose tolerance factor (GTF) which has a role as a cofactor to insulin. GTF is also released into circulation following glucose as does insulin. It helps the binding of insulin to tissue receptor sites. Thus, it is essential for insulin action. In the deficiency of chromium or GTF, glucose removal from blood is decreased. People in old age, seems to suffer from chromium deficiency, because chromium supplementation in the diet have helped to improve their tolerance to glucose. Chromium is also reported to lower blood cholesterol levels. Normal diet meets the chromium requirements. Chromium deficiency in experimental animals also results in growth reduction.

Summary

The summary of functions, dietary sources and deficiency of various minerals is given in Table 5.4.

Table 5.4: Summary of functions, dietary sources and deficiency symptoms of various minerals

Minerals	Functions	Dietary sources	Deficiency symptoms
Macroelements			
Sodium	Plasma volume, nerve and muscles function; extracellular cation	Common salt	Deficiency unknown, excess leads to hypertension in susceptible individuals
Potassium	Nerve and muscles function, intracellular cation	Fruits, nuts	Muscular weakness, mental confusion, excess leads to cardiac arrest
Chloride	Fluid and electrolyte balance	Common salt	Primary deficiency unknown; secondary deficiency due to diarrhoea, vomiting
Calcium	Constituent of bone and teeth; muscles and nerve function	Dairy products, beans, leafy vegetables	Parathesias, muscular excitability, cramps, bone fracture
Phosphorous	Constituent of bone and teeth, phosphoproteins	Dairy products	Deficiency is rare, secondary hypophosphatemia leads to skeletal deformities
Magnesium	Constituent of bone and teeth, enzyme cofactor	Green leafy vegetables	Neuromuscular excitability, cramps, parathesias
Microelements			
Iron	Components of heme, iron sulphur protein	Red meat, liver, eggs	Anemia; excess leads to hemochromatosis
Iodine	Component of thyroid hormones	Iodized salt, sea food enzymes	Goiter
Copper	Component of oxidases enzymes	Liver	Anemia
Zinc	Enzyme cofactor	Meat, liver, eggs	Hypogonadism, impairment in growth, wound healing, sense of taste and smell
Fluorine	Normal and strong bones and teeth	Sea food, tea and drinking water	Dental caries; excess leads to fluorosis
Chromium	Cofactor for insulin	Brewer's yeast, spices	Glucose intolerance

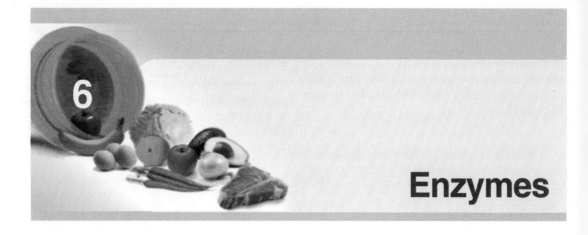

6

Enzymes

INTRODUCTION

You might have wondered as to how the reactions occur so fast in living organisms, the answer is because of enzymes. Enzymes are proteins which catalyze the reactions in biological systems. Both the enzymes and the catalysts have same salient features:

1. They are effective in small amount.
2. They are unchanged at the end of the reaction.
3. They do not affect the equilibrium of a reversible chemical reaction.
4. They exhibit specificity in its ability to catalyze chemical reaction.

The last mentioned feature is much more marked in case of enzymes because many enzymes exist in the cell and they have to act at the same time.

The enzymes are very efficient. The efficiency of enzymes can be imagined by an example of catalase enzyme. One mg of this enzyme produces 2740 liters of oxygen per hour at 0°C.

$$2H_2O_2 \xrightarrow{\text{Catalase}} 2H_2O + O_2$$

As a catalyst, the enzymes lower the activation energy of a chemical reaction. The compound on which enzyme acts is called substrate. The name of enzyme is generally termed by putting suffix-ase to the name of substrates. Active site is the part of the enzyme molecule to which substrate combines.

$$A \xrightarrow{E} S \qquad \text{Maltose} \xrightarrow{\text{Maltase}} 2 \text{ Glucose}$$

Almost all the life processes are mediated by enzymes. For example, digestion, absorption, metabolism, intracellular oxidation—reduction, blood coagulation, calcification, detoxication and muscle contraction, all require the participation of enzymes. Thus, it has been rightly said that "the life may be regarded as a cooperating system of an array of enzymatic reactions."

CLASSIFICATION

International Union of Biochemistry (IUB) appointed an Enzyme Commission (EC) which systematically classified all enzymes and identified each enzyme by specific numbers, e.g. 1.3.5.9. Broadly all enzymes have been classified into six major classes and the first number of enzyme denotes the class to which it belongs. Second and third number represents type of reaction within the class in terms of the chemical groups involved. The fourth is the number of the particular enzyme. We here show the six major classes of enzyme classification proposed by IUB.

1. **Oxido-reductases:** Catalyze oxidation–reduction reactions.

$$\text{Lactic acid + NAD} \xrightarrow{\text{Lactate dehydrogenase}} \text{Pyruvic acid + NADH}_2$$

Some sub-classes of oxido-reductase are:

a. *Oxidases:* Catalyze reaction of molecular oxygen

b. *Oxygenases:* Catalyze incorporations of molecular oxygen into substrate.

c. *Oxidative deaminases:* Catalyze the oxidation of amino compounds with formation of ammonia.

d. *Hydroxylases:* Catalyze the introduction of hydroxyl radical into the substrate.

e. *Peroxidases:* Act on hydrogen peroxide.

2. **Transferases:** Catalyze transfer of functional groups (other than hydrogen).

Acetyl CoA + Choline $\xrightarrow{\text{Choline acyltransferase}}$
CoA + Acetylcholine

For example:

a. *Aminotransferases:* Catalyze exchange of amino and keto group between amino and keto acids.

b. *Kinases:* Catalyze the reaction of phosphate radicals.

c. *Glycosyltransferases:* Catalyze the transfer of glycosyl groups.

3. **Hydrolases:** Catalyze hydrolysis reactions. All digestive enzymes belong to this category.

Sucrose + H_2O $\xrightarrow{\text{Sucrase}}$ Glucose + Fructose

A number of hydrolases are present for example:

a. *Peptidases:* Catalyze hydrolyses of peptide bonds.

b. *Glycosidases:* Catalyze hydrolyses of glycosidic bonds.

c. *Esterases:* Catalyze hydrolyses of carboxylic acid esters.

d. *Phosphatases:* Catalyze hydrolyses of phosphoric acid esters.

e. *Phosphodiesterases:* Catalyze hydrolyses of phosphodiester bonds.

f. *Deamidases:* Catalyze hydrolyses of amides.

4. **Lyases:** Note that lysis means breakdown, so lyases catalyze breaking of bonds, like, C–C, C–O, C–N, C–S bond.

Fructose1, 6-diphosphate $\xrightarrow{\text{Aldolase}}$
Glyceraldehyde-3-phosphate +
Dihydroxyacetonephosphate

For example, aldolase catalyzes breaking of C–O bond of the substrate.

5. **Isomerases:** Catalyze interconversion of different isomers. For example:

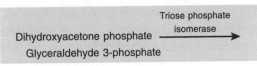

Dihydroxyacetone phosphate $\xrightarrow{\substack{\text{Triose phosphate}\\\text{isomerase}}}$
Glyceraldehyde 3-phosphate

Subclasses

a. *Racemases:* Catalyze the interconversion of D and L isomers and *vice versa* of a compound.

b. *Epimerases:* Catalyze the formation of an epimer of the substrate.

c. *Cis-trans isomerases:* Catalyze the interconversion of the cis-trans isomers of the substrate.

d. *Aldolase-ketoses isomerases:* Catalyze the conversion of aldose to ketose and *vice versa.*

e. *Mutases:* Catalyze the intermolecular transfer of a group.

6. **Ligases (or synthetases):** Catalyze linking/binding together of two compounds with ATP cleavage (to supply energy to drive the reaction).

Examples:

Glutamate + NH_3 + ATP $\xrightarrow{\text{Glutamine synthetase}}$
Glutamine + ADP + PP

Note that "ligase" means "to bind" and that hydrolysis of ATP or a similar high energy compound supplies energy needed to complete the synthesis.

a. *Synthetases:* Catalyze the formation of C–O, C–S, C–N bonds at the expense of energy.

b. *Carboxylases:* Catalyze the introduction of carboxyl group with a C-C bond formation at the expenses of ATP.

In order to remember the six classes in correct order, the word "OTHLIL" may be memorized. It indicates first letter of each group in sequence.

Nomenclature

A vast number of enzymes exist in the cell. A few examples of how the names of enzymes are derived is given below-

a. **On the basis of name of the substrate acted upon by the enzyme:** By adding suffix 'ase' in the name of substrate catalyzed, e.g. lipase, sucrase, maltase, etc.

b. **On the basis of type of reaction catalyzed:** By adding suffix 'ase' in the name of reaction catalyzed, e.g. hydrolase, isomerase, oxidase, dehydrogenase, transaminase, etc.

c. **On the basis of substrate acted upon and reaction catalyzed:** It is virtually the combination of (A) and (B). First the name of the substrate is written and then by adding suffix 'ase' in the type of reaction catalyzed. For example, succinate dehydrogenase, L-glutamic dehydrogenase, etc.

Specificity of Enzymes

One of the most important characteristics of enzymes is the specificity. Enzymes are much more specific in their action as compared to catalysts. Specificity is the property of enzymes by virtue of which one enzyme acts on only one substrate or a very limited number of structurally related substrates. It is this property or specificity which makes it possible for a vast number of enzymes to co-exist in the cell without interfering in each other's actions. Specificity was likened to "the key to a lock" by Emil Fisher. The following four types of specificity have been recognized.

1. **Absolute specificity:** Certain enzymes will act on only one substrate and catalyze one particular reaction. Thus, they show absolute specificity. Urease is such an enzyme.

$$\text{Urea} \xrightarrow{\text{Urease}} \text{Ammonia}$$

2. **Stereochemical specificity:** Some enzymes show stereochemical specificity, i.e. they act on only one type of stereoisomer. For example, L-lactic acid dehydrogenase will act only on L-lactic acid and not D-lactic acid, although the two molecules are mirror image of each other.

$$
\begin{array}{cc}
\text{CH}_3 & \text{CH}_3 \\
| & | \\
\text{HO} - \text{C} - \text{H} & \text{H} - \text{C} - \text{OH} \\
| & | \\
\text{COOH} & \text{COOH} \\
\text{L-lactic acid} & \text{D-lactic acid}
\end{array}
$$

3. **Linkage specificity:** Many enzymes are linkage specific, i.e. they require particular linkage or bond to act upon; the nature of other groups is immaterial. Esterases and lipases are linkage specific enzymes. Esterases hydrolyze ester bond formed between acid and alcohol irrespective of their nature. Similarly, lipase hydrolyze ester bond formed by combination of glycerol with any fatty acid.

4. **Group specificity:** Most of the enzymes come under this category. Group specific enzymes require the presence of a particular linkage as well as certain additional groups before they act. The proteolytic enzymes are group specific enzymes. For example, chymotrypsin preferentially hydrolyzes centrally located peptide bonds in which the carboxylic group is contributed by aromatic amino acids.

FACTORS AFFECTING ENZYME ACTIVITY

There are numerous factors or conditions which affect the enzyme activity. These are discussed below.

1. **Concentration of enzyme:** In order to study the effect of varying enzyme con-

centration on the rate of reaction, it is determined at different enzyme concentrations while keeping the substrate concentration constant. As shown in Fig. 6.1 at zero enzyme concentration, the rate of reaction is also zero. On increasing enzyme concentration, the reaction rate increases proportionately as evidenced by a straight line.

2. **Concentration of substrate:** The rate of reaction is determined at different concentrations of the substrate while keeping enzyme concentration constant. This time, a different type of curve (Fig. 6.2) is obtained. It can be seen that at zero substrate concentration, the rate of reaction is also zero; it rapidly increases on increasing the concentration of substrate. The curve then attains a plateau showing that there is no more increase in the reaction rate on further increase in the substrate concentration. However, the reaction rate can be increased by increasing the enzyme concentration. This indicates that enzyme and substrate combine to form a complex (enzyme-substrate complex or activated complex) and when the entire enzyme is complexed with substrate, the plateau of the curve is obtained. Uncatalyzed reactions do not show such saturation effect.

3. **Temperature:** The temperature is very important factor determining the rate of reaction. The rise in temperature undoubtedly increases the rate of reaction but at the same time, it also denatures the enzyme protein. Therefore, there is a temperature at which the reaction rate is maximum. It is called optimum temperature; on either side of this temperature, the reaction rate decreases (Fig. 6.3). For most of the enzymes, the optimum temperature is around the normal body temperature. Thus, at body temperature, the enzymes are effective maximally. Any rise in body temperature as occurs in fevers will lower the reaction rate of cellular enzymes.

4. **pH:** The pH or hydrogen ion concentration of the medium also affects the enzymatic activity. This is quite expected

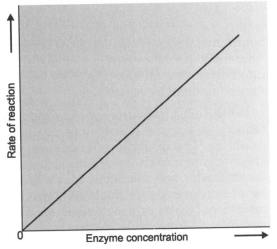

Fig. 6.1: Effect of enzyme concentration

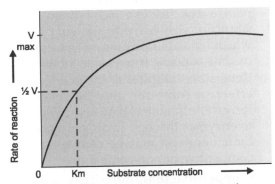

Fig. 6.2: Effect of substrate concentration

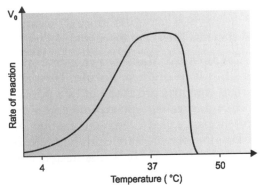

Fig. 6.3: Effect of temperature

because enzymes are proteins and pH affects the state of ionization of the groups present at the active site (*see* mechanism). If the reaction rate is plotted against pH, a "bell-shaped" curve is obtained (Fig. 6.4). The highest enzymatic activity is observed at a pH which is called optimum pH, and the enzyme activity gradually diminishes on both sides of this pH.

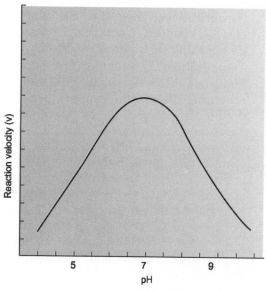

Fig. 6.4: Effect of pH

For most of the enzymes, the pH optimum is around neutrality which corresponds to intracellular pH. However, certain enzymes act at extreme pH—pepsin (pH 2), alkaline phosphatase (pH 10).

Apart from these four general factors, some enzymes activity is affected by various substances. These are discussed below.

Coenzymes: Many enzymes are made up of only protein molecule. However, certain enzymes are made of two parts—a protein part called apoenzyme and a non-protein part called coenzyme; neither part possess the enzyme activity individually but the enzymatic activity is manifested when both the parts combine.

Holoenzyme = Apoenzyme + Coenzyme

A coenzyme is regarded as a co-substrate. It is non-protein, heat stable and dialyzable organic compound. In fact, the vitamins of B-complex group, after suitable transformation in the body, act as coenzyme of some enzyme. The oxidoreductases and transferases are enzymes which usually belong to this category. In absence of particular B-complex vitamin, the relevant coenzyme is not formed affecting catalysis of that particular reaction.

Activators: Sometimes the activity of enzymes is affected by addition or presence of certain compounds which are called modifiers. Activators are positive modifiers of the enzymatic activity. They are usually the metal ions. Some enzymes, like alcohol dehydrogenase (Zn^{2+}), xanthine oxidase (Fe^{3+}, Mo^{4+}) and hexokinase (Mg^{2+}) contain highly reproducible number of tightly bound metal ions per molecule of protein. The removal of these metal ions often results into partial or total loss of activity, which may be restored by replacing it.

Inhibitors: If addition of a compound reduces the enzyme activity, it is called the inhibitor. The inhibition of enzymes by specific compounds is very important in Biochemistry and Medicine. Many drugs have been developed on this basis of enzyme inhibition. Two types of inhibition have been recognized—irreversible and reversible.

a. **Irreversible inhibitors** bind covalently to enzyme and cause permanent inactivation. Examples are toxic organophosphorus insecticides which bind to active site of acetylcholine esterase, and cyanide which binds to iron atom of cytochrome oxidase, causing irreversible inhibition.

b. **Reversible inhibitor** is one in which the effect of inhibitor may be reversed. Reversible inhibitors bind non-covalently to enzymes through hydrogen bonds or ionic bonds. It may be of two types—competitive or non-competitive.

Competitive inhibitors: They compete with substrate for active site of enzyme for binding. The inhibitor has structure similar to the substrate so it binds at active site of enzyme, thus, preventing the binding of substrate in that place with the result that no reaction takes place (Fig. 6.5a). However, the competitive inhibition can be reversed by increasing substrate concentration sufficiently. Sulfanilamide and other sulfa drugs have structure similar to p-amino-benzoic acid (PABA), hence, they act as competitive inhibitors to the enzyme of bacteria which synthesize folic acid (which is essential for their growth) from PABA. This is precisely how sulfa drugs stop the bacterial growth. Other example of drugs acting as enzyme inhibitors is allopurinol in gout (inhibits enzyme xanthine oxidase) and methotrexate in cancer (inhibits dihydro-folate reductase).

H₂N— ⟨benzene ring⟩ —COOH   H₂N— ⟨benzene ring⟩ —SO₂HN
    PABA   Sulfanilamide

Non-competitive inhibitors: The inhibitor has no structural resemblance with the substrate. It binds to the enzyme at a site other than active site. This causes distortion in the three dimensional structure of enzyme which results into inhibition of enzyme activity (Fig. 6.5b).

Heavy metal ions, like Hg^{2+}, Pb^{2+} act as inhibitors of enzymes containing free SH-groups by combining with these groups which alter enzymes activity.

Allosteric Enzymes

Enzymes having two or more subunits have a catalytic site, also called as a regulatory site or the allosteric site which is different than the active site. Both the sites are located on different subunits of the enzyme. Such enzymes are called allosteric enzyme or regulatory enzyme. These enzymes are regulated by certain substances called allosteric modulators (effectors) which reversibly bind to the enzyme at the allosteric site.

An interaction with the effector molecule brings about conformational changes in the catalytic site of the enzyme. The binding of the effector molecule may result in the inhibition of the enzymatic action (allosteric inhibition). Such an effector molecule is called a negative effector (allosteric inhibitor). On the other hand, an effector may activate the enzymatic reaction (allosteric activation) and is called a positive effector (allosteric activator). For example, isocitrate dehydrogenase which controls citric acids cycle, is an allosteric enzyme. This enzyme is allosterically activated by ADP and inhibited by ATP.

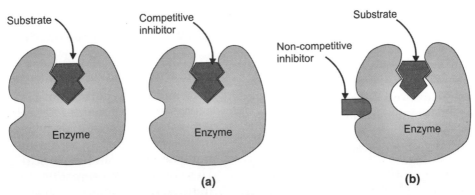

(a)   (b)

Fig. 6.5: Mechanism of action of (a) competitive and (b) non-competitive inhibitors

MECHANISM OF ENZYME ACTION

The exact mechanism of action of individual enzymes differs. However, certain general features of mechanism of enzyme action are considered here.

1. Enzymes have molecular weight in the range of 10^4 to 10^6 while substrates in the range of 10^2 to 10^3. Thus, enzymes are 100 to 1000 times larger than the substrates.
2. The enzymes lower the energy of activation (Fig. 6.6).
3. The active site is that part of the enzyme with which the substrate is actually bound. The part of the enzyme molecule not in physical contact with the substrate but function in the catalytic process is known as catalytic site.
4. The active site takes up a relatively small part of the total volume of an enzyme.
5. The substrate is bound to enzyme by relatively weak forces.

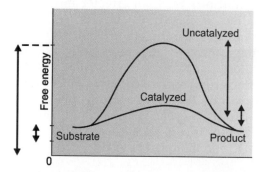

Fig. 6.6: Decrease in activation energy by enzyme

Based on these generalizations, two theories have been proposed to explain their mechanism of action. These are similar to those for catalysts in inorganic chemistry.

a. Physical adsorption theory
b. Chemical combination theory.

Physical Adsorption Theory

This theory suggests that substrate molecules are adsorbed on the surface of enzyme molecule. This view is supported by large size of enzyme molecule as compared to substrate where physical adsorption is expected to play a role. Physical proximity of reactants may increase collisions between molecules. The fact that the enzyme lowers the energy of activation of a reaction also supports this theory.

$$A + B \xrightarrow{\;E\;} C + D$$

Chemical Combination Theory

This theory suggests that enzymes actually take part in the reactions.

$$E + S \longrightarrow \underset{\text{Activated complex}}{ES} \longrightarrow P + E$$

The chemical combination between substrate and enzyme is supported by following evidences.

1. X-ray crystallographic, electron microscopic and spectroscopic examination of enzyme and substrate during catalysis show changes in the enzyme structure with progress of reaction.
2. The curve of the rate of reaction *versus* substrate concentration with a fixed concentration of enzyme (Fig. 6.2) also supports enzyme substrate complex (ES) formation because if the substrate and enzyme did not combine, the curve would have been a straight line.

Thus, regarding enzyme catalysis, the two theories seem to be complementary rather than contradictory.

ENZYME ACTIVITY VERSUS ITS SPECIFICITY

Two views have been proposed to relate enzyme activity and the specificity.

1. **Lock and key hypothesis of Fisher:** The active site is considered as a rigid template and compounds with complementary structure to active site would combine, just as 'key fits a lock' (Fig. 6.7a). This also explains competitive inhibition.
2. **Induced fit hypothesis of Koshland:** The binding of substrate to enzyme can bring

about conformational changes to make the active site exactly complementary to the substrate molecule. This may be likened to the shape of a glove when a hand is inserted (Fig. 6.7b).

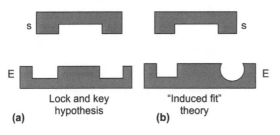

(a) Lock and key hypothesis   (b) "Induced fit" theory

Fig. 6.7: Theories of mechanism of enzyme action

DIAGNOSTIC IMPORTANCE OF BLOOD ENZYMES

With the lysis of cells, the intracellular enzymes are released into blood. So certain amount of them is always present in it. This is called normal blood level of enzyme. This normal level rises by increased rate of production due to abnormal or increased breakdown of cells owing to disease processes. The increased blood level of certain enzymes has clinical significance. It helps the clinician in diagnosis.

Given below is the list of enzymes more commonly determined in clinical bio-

chemistry laboratory and their significance in relation to diagnosis of diseases (Table 6.1).

The enzyme estimation is particularly useful in the diagnosis of heart attack or myocardial infarction. The enzyme CPK significantly rises within 4–8 hours of infarction so with its help, MI can be detected as early as that. On the other hand, LDH remains elevated much longer in blood, so it can be used to detect MI as late as 7–8 days. Similarly, in acute viral hepatitis, there is a rapid rise in the level of transaminase (GPT), much before rise in bilirubin level or appearance of jaundice.

ISOENZYMES

'Iso' means 'same', hence, literally isoenzyme means same enzyme. Just as we have isotopes of an element which have same chemical properties, there are isoenzymes which catalyze same chemical reaction. Previously it was believed that there is one enzyme protein to catalyze one reaction. Now it is recognized that there is more than one enzyme protein catalyzing a reaction. So in the simplest words, isoenzymes may be defined as "different proteins with similarly enzymatic activity." Isoenzymes differ in

Table 6.1: Some common enzymes in blood	
Enzymes	Diseases in which enzyme is raised
Amylase	Mumps, acute pancreatitis
Acid phosphatase	Cancer prostate
AST or GOT (glutamate oxaloacetate transaminase)	Myocardial infarction
LDH (lactate dehydrogenase)	Viral hepatitis
ALP (alkaline phophatase)	Fracture, infective hepatitis, obstructive jaundice
Gamma-glutamyl transpeptidase	Alcoholic cirrhosis
Creatine phosphokinase	Myocardial infarction, muscles diseases

physical, chemical and immunological properties but catalyze same reaction with different efficiency.

LDH was the first enzyme found to exist in various forms (LDH_1, LDH_2, LDH_3, LDH_4 and LDH_5). Now about a thousand enzymes are known to exist in more than one form. These forms may be present in different tissues or in the same tissue. Occasionally, isoenzymes are distributed differently in different tissues.

LDH isoenzymes: It is a tetramer made up of different combination of two polypeptide chains H and M type which stand for heart and muscle, respectively. The five different forms are:

LDH_1–H_4	LDH_2–H_3M
LDH_3–H_2M_2	LDH_4–HM_3
LDH_5–M_4	

The isoenzymes of LDH have immense value in diagnosis of heart and liver diseases. Increased level of LDH_1 is indicative of myocardial infarction; it increases within 12–24 hours of infarction and persists in circulation for about a week. LDH_5 is increased in diseases of muscles.

CPK isoenzymes: The other enzyme whose isoenzymes have been studied very well is CPK (creatine phosphokinase), also known as creatine kinase (CK). The enzyme is a dimer, made of two polypeptide chains—B (brain) and M (muscle) types. It exists in three distinct forms.

CPK_1–BB–Present in brain
CPK_2–MB–Present in heart
CPK_3–MM–Present in skeletal muscle

In healthy individuals, CPK_2 fraction is less than 2% of total CPK activity in plasma. It is raised several times in myocardial infarction. It is the earliest change occurring in blood in this disease, is very reliable and quite sensitive, so its determination in heart diseases is preferred over other parameters.

ALP isoenzymes: The enzymes, alkaline phosphate (ALP) are also present in several forms. They contain same proteins but only differ in their content of sialic acid (a carbohydrate). In normal healthy person, only two forms are observed in serum. These are ALP_1 which comes from liver and ALP_2 which originates from the bone. Any rise in the either fraction denotes the disease of that particular organ.

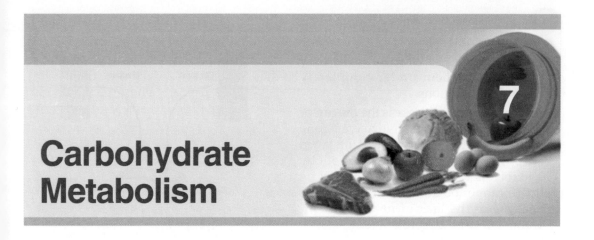

Carbohydrate Metabolism

7

INTRODUCTION

The carbohydrates are major source of energy for most of the persons partly because of stability of plant food and partly because it is relatively less expensive. The important dietary carbohydrates are—glucose, fructose, galactose, pentose, sucrose, lactose, maltose, starch and dextrin, but glucose is by far the most important nutrient and metabolite.

Metabolism describes the chemical changes that are constantly taking place in the billions of cells that make up the living body. Anabolism means synthesis; catabolism means breakdown. Generally, anabolism consumes energy while catabolism liberates energy. Metabolism is preceded by digestion and absorption. A summarized view of carbohydrate metabolism is given in Fig. 7.1.

The central theme in the above scheme is 'blood sugar' which is maintained at a constant level (80–120 mg%). It is necessary to maintain this level for following reasons:

1. **Brain and nervous system:** These utilize only glucose for energy. Severe hypoglycemia may lead to brain dysfunction, coma and finally death.

2. **Erythrocytes:** RBCs also use glucose as the only fuel for energy.

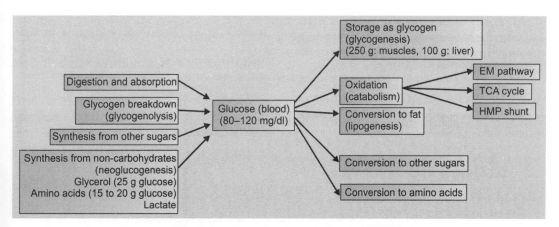

Fig. 7.1: View of carbohydrate metabolism

3. **Skeletal muscles:** Glucose is the only fuel used by them under completely anaerobic conditions.

4. **Adipose tissue:** Glucose is the precursor of glycerol moiety (dihydroxyacetone phosphate) for the synthesis of fat in adipose tissue. Glycerol formed by hydrolysis of fat in adipose tissue by lipase cannot be utilized for resynthesis because of the lack of necessary activating enzyme, glycerokinase.

5. **Mammary glands:** Lactating mammary glands need glucose to synthesize lactose.

6. **All tissues:** A minimum amount of glucose is needed by all tissues to replenish the intermediates of TCA cycle and to completely oxidize fatty acids.

The normal blood sugar level is maintained by a number of processes. The processes shown in the left side in Fig. 7.1 add sugar to the blood while processes shown on the right side remove glucose from the blood. Normally there is a balance between the two processes so that blood glucose level is maintained within normal limits as required (Fig. 7.2).

The most important process which adds glucose to the blood is the digestion and absorption of dietary carbohydrates. When this process is over, glucose is contributed by the breakdown of glycogen in liver. Since this capacity is limited, glucose is synthesized from non-carbohydrate sources (called neoglucogenesis). On the other side, the most important process which removes glucose from blood is oxidation in tissues to provide energy. After meeting the energy needs of the body, remaining glucose is converted into glycogen or fat and stored for future use.

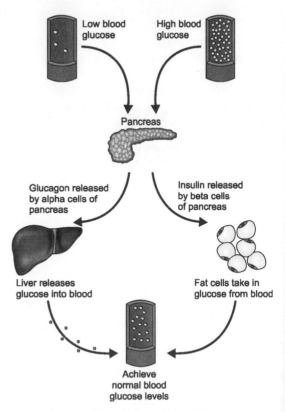

Fig. 7.2: Regulation of blood glucose

DIGESTION AND ABSORPTION

The digestion and absorption of carbohydrates occur in the gastrointestinal tract.

Carbohydrate digestion starts in the mouth by the salivary amylase (also called ptyalin) but is relatively unimportant because of very short time, food remains in the mouth. Salivary amylase is readily inactivated at pH below 4.0 which is found in the stomach. Some of the sucrose present get hydrolyzed by the action of HCl. The carbohydrates are mainly digested in intestine by pancreatic α-amylase.

Pancreatic α-amylase (pH-7.1) converts starch, dextrin and glycogen into maltose and isomaltase by hydrolyzing α-1, 4-linkages. α-1, 6 bonds are hydrolyzed by α-dextrinase (oligo-1, 6-hydrolase).

Starch, dextrin and glycogen $\xrightarrow{\alpha\text{-amylase}}$ Maltose + Isomaltose

Mucosal cells of duodenum and jejunum contain several disaccharides which hydrolyze specific disaccharides. Hydrolysis occurs within the cells. The pictorial presentation of digestion of carbohydrate is given in Fig. 7.3. The resulting monosaccharides are transferred from the cells into the blood.

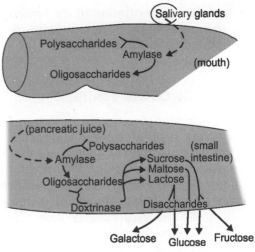

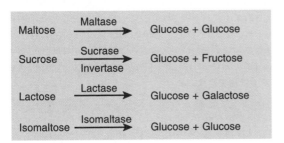

Fig. 7.3: Digestion of carbohydrates

Cellulose is not digested in human gut due to the absence of cellulase which acts on β-1, 4 linkages, hence it is passed in the stool as its bulk.

Carbohydrate absorption occurs in proximal small intestine, i.e. duodenum and jejunum. Absorption rates of monosaccharide differ because different monosaccharides are absorbed by different mechanisms. The rate of absorption is highest for galactose and glucose. Glucose and galactose are absorbed by active transport, which occurs against concentration gradient and requires a carrier, energy from ATP and co-transport of Na^+ (Fig. 7.4). Hence, the absorption rate is independent of sugar concentration. Other sugars are transported by simple diffusion

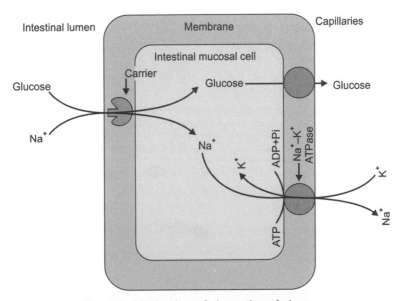

Fig. 7.4: Mechanism of absorption of glucose

from higher concentration in the lumen to lower concentration in blood. Fructose is transported by facilitated diffusion.

GLYCOGEN SYNTHESIS

The structure of glycogen is very complex. It is a very high molecular weight compound. It is made up of a large number of glucose units, i.e. about 25000 units. Its structure is highly branched. The branching occurs after 8–12 units. Branching increases solubility. The structure is like a tree (Fig. 7.5). General formula of glycogen may be written as $(C_6H_{11}O_5)$ n or $(Glucose)_n$. Thus, it is a glucose monomer.

Glycogen occurs in most mammalian cells, but stored in liver and muscles. In muscles, its concentration is less than 2%. Liver concentration varies from 5 to 10% on feeding and down to 0.1% after 24 hrs. fasting. Thus, liver glycogen is much more labile and is an effective store of immediately available energy. It functions as a store of glucose.

The details of glycogen synthesis are given below.

- UDP: uridine diphosphate
- UTP: uridine triphosphate
- UDPG: uridine diphosphate glucose
- PPi: released pyrophosphate
- Pi: inorganic phosphate

Details of Synthesis of Glycogen (Glycogenesis)

The synthesis occurs mainly in liver and muscle. For this purpose, the glucose molecule has to be first activated by phosphorylation and then the glucose moieties are transferred to UTP (uridine triphosphate) which acts as a donor of glucose to growing chain. First the straight chain is established. For establishing branching, a segment of straight chain is removed and reattached by alpha 1,6-linkage. The net reaction may be represented as:

$$(Glucose)_n + UDP\ Glucose \longrightarrow (Glucose)_{n+1} + UDP$$

The individual steps are given below:

1. Phosphorylation of glucose

$$Glucose \xrightarrow[\substack{ATP \quad ADP}]{Hexokinase} Glucose\text{-}6\text{-}phosphate$$

2. Conversion of G-6-P to G-1-P

$$G\text{-}6\text{-}P \underset{glucomutase}{\overset{Phospho}{\longleftrightarrow}} G\text{-}1\text{-}P$$

3. Transfer of glucose to UTP

$$G\text{-}1\text{-}P + UTP \xrightarrow{\substack{Glucose\text{-}1\text{-}phosphate \\ uridyl\ transferase}}$$

UDPG   +   PPi
Uridine diphosphate   Pyrophosphate
glucose

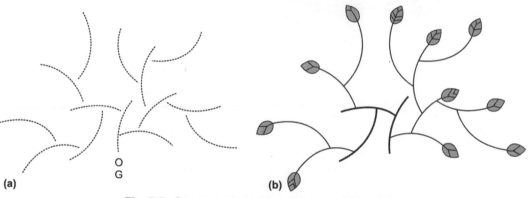

Fig. 7.5: Structure of glycogen (a), resembles tree (b)

4. Addition of glucose to growing glycogen chain by α-1, 4 linkage

UDPG   + (Glucose)$_n$+ $\xrightarrow{\text{Glycogen Synthetase}}$

(Glucose)$_{n+1}$ +   UDP

G–G–G–G + UDPG $\longrightarrow$
G–G–G–G–G   +   UDP

5. Establishment of branching

When the chain has been lengthened to 7–8 residues, a branching enzyme acts. It removes a section of already formed chain and reattaches to the same or to a neighboring chain by α-1, 6 bonds to create proper branching.

Thus, by repetitive action of glycogen synthetase and branching enzyme, the glycogen molecule (Fig. 7.5) is formed.

GLYCOGEN BREAKDOWN (GLYCOGENOLYSIS)

Glycogenolysis means the lysis or breakdown of glycogen. In the liver, glycogen is not broken down by hydrolysis as occurs during its digestion in gut. On the contrary, glycogen is first cleaved by an enzyme, phosphorylase which catalyzes the following reaction

(Glycogen)$_{n+1}$ + Pi = (Glycogen)$_n$ +
Glucose-1-phosphate

and then by a debranching enzyme (as indicated in Fig. 7.6) which liberates free glucose from branch points (α-1, 6-bonds). The sum total of these reactions is:

Glycogen + n H$_3$PO$_4$ ↔ n–Glucose-1-P (90%) + X Glucose (10%)

The steps of glycogenolysis are shown in Fig. 7.6:

1. Action of phosphorylase: The first step of glycogen breakdown is the sequential phosphorylation of glucose units joined by α-1, 4-glycosidic bonds by *glycogen phosphorylase*. This enzyme only splits α-1, 4 links and is unable to act between branch points.

2. Action of debranching enzyme: This enzyme first transfers a piece of α-1, 4 chains from one of the chain to another chain, leaving a single glucose residue linked by α-1, 6 bonds. Then this single glucose linked by α-1, 6-linkage is removed as a free glucose molecule.

3. Action of phosphorylase: Phosphorylase now again attacks the remaining α-1, 4-linked chain. Thus, by the combined action of the phosphorylase and debranching enzymes, 90% of glucose-1-phosphate and 10% of glucose are produced.

4. Action of phosphoglucomutase: It converts glucose-1-phosphate into glycose-6-phosphate.

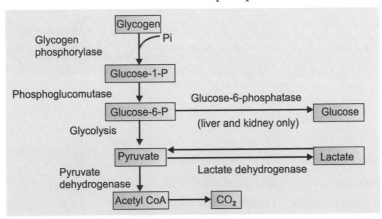

Fig. 7.6: Glycogenolysis

$$G-1-\text{\textcircled{P}} \underset{\text{glucomutase}}{\overset{\text{Phospho}}{\rightleftharpoons}} G-6-\text{\textcircled{P}}$$

5. **Fate of glucose-6-phosphate:** Liver contains an enzyme glucose-6-phosphatase, which gives free glucose so that liver glycogen can serve as a source of glucose to the blood. However, this enzyme is absent in muscle so the muscle glycogen does not contribute to blood glucose, but of glucose-6-phosphate whose fate (further utilization) is shown below.

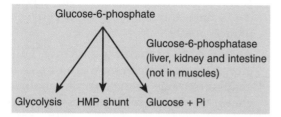

Glycogen Storage Diseases

The biosynthesis and breakdown of glycogen is so important that hereditary absence of any of the enzyme results in the disease. These are called glycogen storage disease (Table 7.1). Generally these deficiencies lead to excessive accumulation of glycogen and/or inability to use that glycogen as a fuel source.

FATE OF ABSORBED MONOSACCHARIDES

Most of the monosaccharides (galactose, fructose, etc.) are metabolized after their conversion into glucose so the metabolism of carbohydrate is mainly the metabolism of glucose.

The conversion of other sugars into glucose or their independent utilization is shown below.

Utilization of Fructose

Fructose can be utilized by either of the following sequence of reactions and converted into glucose.

a. Fructose + ATP $\xrightarrow{\text{Hexokinase}}$ Fructose-6-phosphate + ADP

b. Fructose-6-phosphate + ATP $\xrightarrow[\text{kinase}]{\text{Phosphofructo-}}$ F-1, 6-P + ADP

c. Fructose-6-phosphate $\underset{\text{PHI}}{\overset{}{\rightleftharpoons}}$ G-6-P

Table 7.1: Glycogen storage diseases

Type	Disease name	Defective enzyme	Glycogen level	Principal tissue affected
I	von Gierke's disease	Glucose-6-phosphatase	High	Liver, kidney
II	Pompe's disease	α-1, 4 glucosidase	Very high	All organs
III	Cori's/Forbes' disease	Debranching enzyme	High	Liver, heart, muscles
IV	Andersen's disease	Branching enzyme	Normal	Liver, spleen, muscles
V	McArdle's disease	Muscle glycogen phosphorylase	High	Muscles
VI	Hers' disease	Liver phosphorylase	High	Liver
VII	Tarui's disease	Phosphofructokinase	High	Muscles
VIII	Hepatic phosphorylase kinase deficiency	Phosphorylase kinase	High	Liver

1. Fructose + ATP $\xrightarrow{\text{Fructokinase}}$

   Fructose-1-phosphate + ADP

2. Fructose-1-phosphate $\xrightarrow[\text{aldolase}]{\text{Fructose-1-phosphate}}$

   Dihydroxyacetone + Glyceralde-
   phosphate   hyde

3. Glyceraldehyde + ATP $\xrightarrow{\text{Kinase}}$

   Glyceraldehyde-3- + ADP
   phosphate

Both these enter glycolytic pathway and metabolized further. Reversal of this would lead to synthesis of glucose.

Utilization of Galactose

Galactose is used for the synthesis of lactose. The biochemical pathway is given below. This scheme also converts galactose into glucose and *vice versa*. Hence, lactose can be synthesized from glucose without needing galactose.

1. Galactose + ATP $\xrightarrow{\text{Galactokinase}}$

   Galactose-1-phosphate + ADP

2. Galactose-1-phosphate + UDP-Glucose

   $\xrightarrow[\text{Uridyl transferase}]{\text{Hexose-1-phosphate}}$ Glucose-1-phosphate + UDP-galactose

3. UDP-galactose $\underset{\text{epimerase}}{\overset{\text{UDP-glucose-4}}{\rightleftharpoons}}$ UDP-glucose

4. UDP-galactose + Glucose $\xrightarrow[\text{synthetase}]{\text{Lactose}}$ Lactose + UDP

Synthesis of lactose occurs in mammary glands by the enzyme lactose synthetase.

Fate of Glucose

After absorption, glucose undergoes either catabolism or anabolism.

1. **Catabolism:** Breakdown or oxidation to yield energy. The pathway is known as glycolysis.

2. **Anabolism:** Anabolic pathway consists of either
   i. Storage as glycogen mainly in muscle and liver, or
   ii. Conversion to fat or amino acids.

GLYCOLYSIS

Glycolysis means breakdown of glucose to yield energy. It is one of the earliest biochemical pathways discovered. In glycolysis, a glucose molecule is converted into pyruvate, then two lactic acid molecules with production of some energy. These reactions do not need oxygen, so the pathway is referred as anaerobic glycolysis. Further breakdown can occur in presence of oxygen to liberate carbon dioxide and water and a large amount of energy. This is called aerobic glycolysis. Aerobic glycolysis yields net 36 molecules of ATP per molecules of glucose, whereas anaerobic glycolysis results in net 2 molecules of ATP generation from one molecule of glucose. Anaerobic glycolysis allows the continued production of ATP in tissue that lacks mitochondria or in cells deprived of sufficient oxygen.

Anaerobic glycolysis: The net reaction of anaerobic glycolysis is:

$$C_6H_{12}O_6 \longrightarrow 2C_3H_6O_3 + 2\,ATP\,(47.0\,kcal/mol)$$
(Glucose)   (Lactic acid)   (Energy)

Aerobic glycolysis: The net reaction of aerobic glycolysis is:

$$C_6H_{12}O_6 \longrightarrow 6CO_2 + 6H_2O + 36\,ATP\,(683.0\,kcal/mol)$$
(Glucose)   (energy)

ANAEROBIC GLYCOLYSIS

It is glucose breakdown in absence of oxygen. Nearly all forms of life utilize anaerobic glycolysis. It is also called Embden Meyerhof (EM) pathway. The flow chart is given in Fig. 7.7 and the steps of anaerobic glycolysis are given in Fig. 7.8, while the individual reactions are discussed after that under the name of enzyme catalyzing the reactions in page 81.

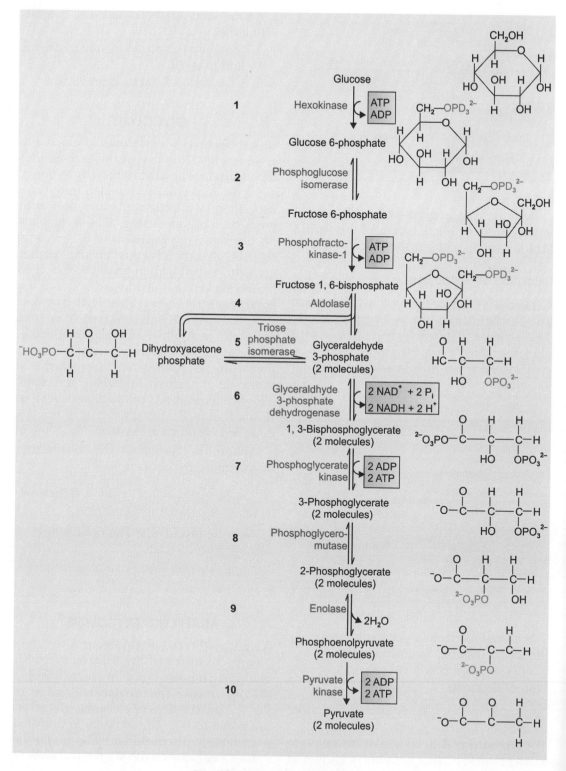

Fig. 7.7: Flow chart of glycolysis

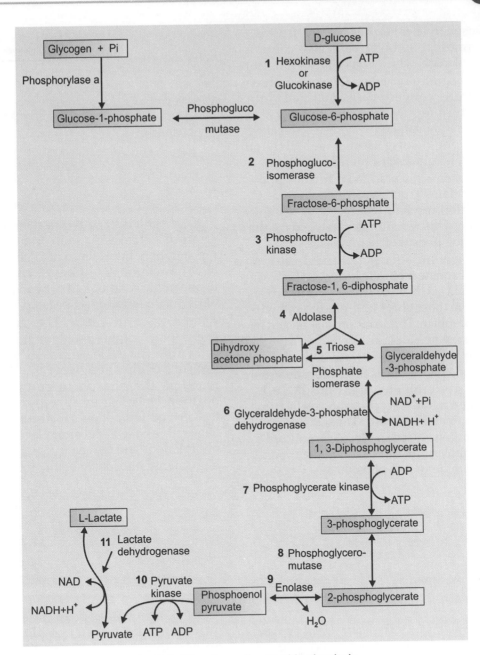

Fig. 7.8: The steps of anaerobic glycolysis

Enzymes Catalyzing Reactions

The conversion of glucose to lactate involves 11 steps. If glycogen is catabolised in this pathway, there are 12 steps.

1. *Hexokinase:* Upon entering the cell, ATP phosphorylates glucose molecule at C_6 to yield glucose-6-phosphate. This reaction is catalyzed by hexokinase or glucokinase. All human cells contain hexokinase which

phosphorylates hexoses-glucose, fructose, mannose, etc. Liver cells also contain glucokinase, which is specific for glucose.

2. *Phosphoglucoisomerase:* Glucose-6-phosphate is converted (isomerized) into fructose-6-phosphate by the enzyme hexose phosphate isomerase also called phospho-hexose isomerase (PHI) or phospho-glucose isomerase (PGI).

3. *Phosphofructokinase:* ATP further phosphorylates fructose-6-phosphate at C_1 position to yield fructose-1, 6-diphosphate. This reaction is catalyzed by the enzyme phosphofructokinase.

4. *Aldolase:* In this reaction fructose-1, 6-diphosphate molecule is cleaved between C_3 and C_4 to form two trioses, dihydroxyacetone phosphate and glyceraldehyde-3-phosphate. This reaction is catalyzed by the enzyme aldolase.

5. *Triose phosphate isomerase:* Dihydroxyacetone phosphate is then interconverted into glyceraldehyde-3-phosphate by isomerization reaction catalyzed by triose phosphate isomerase. Thus, the original six carbon glucose molecule is reduced to two moles of a three carbon compound, glyceraldehyde-3-phosphate.

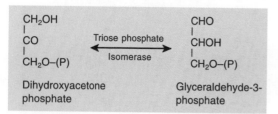

6. *Glyceraldehyde-3-phosphate dehydrogenase:* The overall reaction is the coupling of oxidation to phosphorylation. This reaction is catalyzed by glyceraldehyde-3-phosphate dehydrogenase and requires coenzyme NAD for oxidation and inorganic phosphate for phosphorylation. The energy released by the oxidation of glyceraldehyde-3-phosphate is used for the subsequent phosphorylation of the oxidized product, 3-phosphoglycerate.

CHO
|
CHOH + H_2O + NAD + Pi ⟷ Glyceraldehyde-3-phosphate dehydrogenase
|
CH_2O–(P)

Glyceraldehyde-3-phosphate

COO–(P)
|
CHOH + $NADH_2$
|
CH_2O–(P)

1,3-Diphosphoglycerate

As NAD has been reduced, continuation of glycolysis would require its regeneration. In presence of O_2, it would have been through respiratory chain, but in anaerobic condition, it is by reduction of pyruvate to form lactate (step-11).

7. *Phosphoglycerate kinase:* The chemical energy of 1, 3-diphosphoglycerate is used to synthesize ATP from ADP and to produce 3-phosphoglycerate. In this reaction, the phosphate group at C_1 position of 1, 3-diphosphoglycerate is transferred to another substrate (ADP), hence, it is called "substrate level phosphorylation" and the energy is trapped in high energy phosphate bond of ATP.

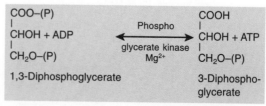

8. *Phosphoglycero mutase:* In this reaction, an intramolecular transfer of phosphate group occurs from C_3 to C_2 when 3-phosphoglycerate is converted into 2-phosphoglycerate by the enzyme phosphoglyceromutase.

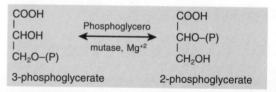

9. *Enolase:* Elimination of an element of H_2O from 2-phosphoglycerate results in the formation of phosphoenol pyruvate which is a very high energy compound. This reaction requires the enzyme called enolase and Mg^{2+} ions.

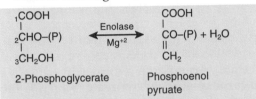

$$\begin{array}{l} {}_1COOH \\ | \\ {}_2CHO–(P) \\ | \\ {}_3CH_2OH \end{array} \quad \underset{Mg^{+2}}{\overset{Enolase}{\rightleftharpoons}} \quad \begin{array}{l} COOH \\ | \\ CO–(P) + H_2O \\ \| \\ CH_2 \end{array}$$

2-Phosphoglycerate   Phosphoenol
                              pyruate

10. *Pyruvate kinase:* The enzyme pyruvate kinase, readily transfers phosphate group from phosphoenol pyruvate to ADP. This is another example of "substrate level phosphorylation". The removal of the phosphate group from phosphoenol pyruvate leaves pyruvate entirely in the keto form. This is very exergonic reaction and is essentially irreversible.

$$\begin{array}{l} COOH \\ | \\ CO–(P) \\ \| \quad + ADP \\ CH_2 \end{array} \quad \underset{Mg^{2+}}{\overset{Pyruvate\ kinase}{\longrightarrow}} \quad \begin{array}{l} COOH \\ | \\ CO \\ | \quad + ATP \\ CH_3 \end{array}$$

Phosphoenol   Pyruvate
pyruvate   (keto form)

11. *Lactate dehydrogenase:* The last step in glycolysis is the reduction of pyruvate to produce lactate by the enzyme, lactate dehydrogenase and coenzyme NADH, which acts as a hydrogen donor. This step is essentially an exercise to regenerate NAD, required for the reaction no. 6, catalyzed by glyceraldehyde-3-phosphate dehydrogenase so that the glycolysis does not stop for want of NAD. It may be noted that the usual way of oxidising NADH by molecular oxygen on ETC is not possible during glycolysis under anaerobic situations.

$$\begin{array}{l} COOH \\ | \\ CO + NADH + H^+ \\ | \\ CH_3 \end{array} \quad \underset{dehydrogenase}{\overset{Lactate}{\rightleftharpoons}} \quad \begin{array}{l} COOH \\ | \\ CHOH + NAD^+ \\ | \\ CH_3 \end{array}$$

Pyruvate   Lactate

Some important points regarding glycolysis are discussed below:

a. The summary of anaerobic glycolysis is expressed in the following equation:

$$\text{Glucose} + 2\ ADP + 2Pi \longrightarrow 2\ \text{lactate} + 2\ ATP + 2H_2O\ (C_3H_6O_3)$$
$$C_6H_{12}O_6$$

b. This pathway occurs in the cytosol or cytoplasmic matrix.

c. There is net production of two moles of ATP per mole of glucose.

d. If glycogen is the source of glucose for glycolysis, then the net synthesis of ATP is 3 moles because no input of ATP is needed to produce glucose-6-phosphate.

e. Since glycolysis is an essential pathway, the systemic lack of one of the eleven glycolytic enzymes is incompatible with life. The persons whose erythrocytes are deficient in one or another glycolytic enzyme, they develop hemolytic anemia, e.g. hemolytic anemias due to deficiency of hexokinase or pyruvate kinase.

f. Essentially irreversible reactions serve as control sites. Three such reactions are those which are catalyzed by hexokinase, phosphofructokinase and pyruvate kinase.

(i) $\text{Glucose} \xrightarrow{\text{Hexokinase}} G–6–P$

(ii) $F–6–P \xrightarrow{\text{Phosphofructokinase}} F-1,6-\text{disphosphate}$

(iii) $\text{Phosphoenol pyruvate} + ADP \xrightarrow{\text{Pyruvate kinase}}$
Pyruvate + ATP

In fact, the rate of glycolysis is essentially controlled by the activity of phosphofructokinase. This allosteric enzyme is stimulated by ADP and AMP and is inhibited by ATP and citrate. In other words, phosphofructokinase is most active when energy charge of a cell is low.

g. Magnesium ion is required by many of the enzymes of glycolysis. Hence, this element has role in utilization of carbohydrates by the body.

Rapaport-Luebering Cycle

In erythrocytes, an alternate pathway of glycolysis occurs in which 1, 3-bisphosphoglycerate (1, 3 BPG) is converted to 2, 3-bisphosphoglycerate instead of 3-bisphosphoglycerate. The enzyme is 2, 3 BPG mutase. 2, 3-bisphosphoglycerate is then converted to 3-phosphoglycerate by phosphatase without releasing ATP as shown below.

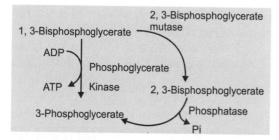

Significance

1. This pathway is operated only in red blood cells when the need for ATP is minimal in RBCs.
2. 2, 3-bisphosphoglycerate enables oxyhemoglobin to unload oxygen to the tissues.

AEROBIC GLYCOLYSIS

The aerobic glycolysis is oxidation of glucose to CO_2 and H_2O, in the presence of oxygen. While anaerobic glycolysis takes place in the cytosol, aerobic oxidation takes place in the mitochondria. It requires the participation of three metabolically interrelated processes—tricarboxylic acid cycle, respiratory chain and oxidative phosphorylation.

Tricarboxylic Acid Cycle

Tricarboxylic acid (TCA) cycle is one of the most important sequence of biochemical reactions which are cyclical in nature. It is also known as Kreb's cycle or citric acid cycle (Fig. 7.9). Now it is known to be a common metabolic pathway for oxidation of all fuel molecules, i.e. carbohydrates, fatty acids (via β-oxidation), glycerol (via E-M pathway) and many amino acids. Apart from energy, it also provides many intermediates for synthesis.

In TCA cycle, oxaloacetate acts as a carrier molecule which is regenerated at the end of the cycle with simultaneous complete oxidation of 2C units (acetyl CoA, active acetate). Acetyl Co A is formed by oxidative decarboxylation of pyruvate (which is the end product of glycolysis).

The steps are discussed here one by one by the name of the enzyme.

1. *Pyruvate dehydrogenase complex:* The formation of acetyl CoA (2C-units) or active acetate is a prerequisite for the entry of the carbon atoms of pyruvate into the TCA cycle. From cytosol, pyruvate rapidly penetrates into mitochondria where it is converted into acetyl coenzyme A (acetyl CoA) by an oxidative decarboxylation reaction that is catalyzed by the pyruvate dehydrogenase complex. The overall reaction is:

$$CH_3-\overset{\overset{\text{O}}{\|}}{C}-COOH + COASH + NAD \longrightarrow CO_2 + NADH_2 + CH_3-\overset{\underset{\text{O}}{\|}}{C}-SCoA$$

Five vitamins, thiamine (TPP), riboflavin (FAD), niacin (NAD), pantothenic acid (CoASH) and lipoic acid participate in this reaction.

2. *Citrate synthase:* Acetyl CoA enters the citric acid cycle by condensing with oxaloacetate to form citrate, a tricarboxylic acid. The reaction is catalyzed by the enzyme citrate synthase. It is essentially irreversible reaction owing to the cleavage of the energy rich thioester linkage in acetyl CoA.

3. *Aconitase:* The isomerisation of citrate to isocitrate is catalyzed by aconitase which contains Fe^{2+}. Aconitase catalyzes hydration and dehydration reactions.

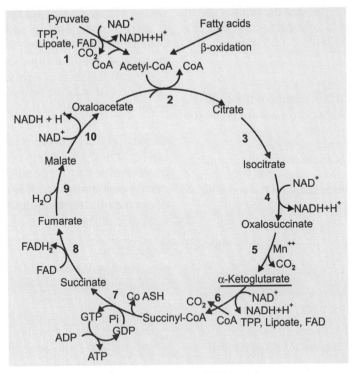

Fig. 7.9: The steps of TCA cycle

4. *and (5) Isocitrate dehydrogenase:* Isocitrate dehydrogenase catalyzes the oxidation and decarboxylation of isocitrate which results in the formation of α-ketoglutarate. This reaction proceeds through the formation of an intermediate oxalosuccinate which remains bound to the enzyme. This oxalosuccinate intermediate results from the oxidation of the hydroxyl group of isocitrate by NAD, and it rapidly undergoes decarboxylation

6. *α-Ketoglutarate dehydrogenase complex:* In a reaction analogous to that catalyzed by the pyruvate dehydrogenase complex, α-ketoglutarate is decarboxylated by α-ketoglutarate dehydrogenase complex, which requires the same five cofactors needed for production of acetyl CoA. The reaction catalyzes the second release of CO_2 in the cycle and the production of succinyl CoA. The overall reaction, like that of the pyruvate dehydrogenase complex, is physiologically irreversible.

7. *Succinate thiokinase:* In the next reaction, succinyl CoA is hydrolyzed to succinate and coenzyme A. The free energy released by the hydrolysis of the thioester bond of succinyl CoA is utilized to synthesize GTP from GDP and Pi. Succinate thiokinase catalyzes this substrate level phosphorylation.

8. *Succinate dehydrogenase:* Succinate is oxidised to yield fumarate by succinate dehydrogenase, which contains a covalently bound FAD molecule that acts as the hydrogen acceptor.

9. *Fumarase:* The addition of water to double bond of fumarate is then catalyzed by fumarase which produces L-malate.

10. *Malate dehydrogenase:* The final step of the cycle is the oxidation of malate, a reaction that is catalyzed by the enzyme malate dehydrogenase requiring NAD as the coenzyme. This reaction regenerates oxaloacetate. The cycle is

now complete and another molecule of oxaloacetate is available to start the cycle.

Notes:

- Oxaloacetate acts as a carrier of the cycle.
- The enzymes of this cycle are found in the mitochondria, closely associated with the enzymes of the respiratory chain.
- Although most of the reactions are reversible, the citrate synthase and α-ketoglutarate dehydrogenase reactions are irreversible.

Summary

From Fig. 7.9, it is apparent that the net effect of the cycle is to oxidise the acetyl group of acetyl CoA to CO_2 with the concomitant reduction of NAD^+ and FAD. Molecular O_2 is not involved in the cycle.

Energetics: The overall reaction for the oxidation of one molecule of pyruvate via the pyruvate dehydrogenase complex and TCA cycle includes the production of three molecules of CO_2, a GTP, four $NADH_2$ and one $FADH_2$. Reduced conezymes $NADH_2$ passes H_2 to respiratory chain in presence of O_2 and generates 3 ATP by oxidative phosphorylation while $FADH_2$ gives only 2 ATP. Thus, we get a total of 15 ATP from one pyruvate molecule. Since glucose produces two molecules of pyruvate, $2 \times 15 = 30$ ATP is produced. To this must be added net production of 2 ATP from glucose molecule in the glycolysis and 6 ATP (2×3 ATP) from oxidation of two moles of lactate through NAD in aerobic conditions. Thus, net production of 38 ATP takes place from one mole of glucose in aerobic glycolysis while output is meager 2 ATP in anaerobic conditions (Table 7.2). Thus, all the fuel molecules (carbohydrates, fats and amino acids) of proteins liberate energy in this manner.

Amphibolic nature: Although TCA cycle is a catabolic pathway which provides a means for the degradation of two carbon acetyl residues that are derived from carbohydrates, fatty acids and amino acids. It also participates in anabolism by providing intermediates for biosynthetic purposes. The intermediates of citric acid cycle are used as a precursor in the biosynthesis of many compounds like glucose from carbon skeleton of amino acids, and providing building blocks for heme synthesis. The TCA cycle is, therefore, amphibolic. Theoretically, one molecule of oxaloacetate should be sufficient to carry the cycle perpetually, but it is not so because of draining of intermediates of TCA cycle for anabolic purposes.

Regulation

a. Citrate synthetase, which is allosterically inhibited by ATP, plays an important role in the regulation of the cycle. When ATP concentration is high, citrate synthase becomes less active and the rate of ATP production from acetyl CoA decreases.

b. Isocitrate dehydrogenase is another important control point in the cycle. This enzyme is allosterically activated by ADP and inhibited by ATP and NADH. Since NADH leads to the generation of ATP, a high concentration of NADH represents a large potential for ATP generation without further functioning of the citric acid cycle. Thus, the NADH and/or NAD are utilized by certain regulatory enzymes as molecular indicators of the energy status of the cell.

Pentose Phosphate Pathway

It is an alternative pathway of glucose catabolism, also known as hexose monophosphate shunt or phospho gluconate pathway (Fig. 7.10). Its site is cytosol of the cell. Its importance is:

1. This pathway does not generate ATP or liberate energy.
2. In this pathway, the synthesis of NADPH occurs which is used for reductive biosynthesis and for furnishing reducing power in biological systems (synthesis of

Table 7.2: Reactions responsible for the generation of ATP during oxidation of glucose

Pathway	Reaction catalyzed by	Method of ~P production	No. of ~P formed per mole of glucose
Glycolysis	Phosphoglycerate kinase	Substrate level	+ 2
	Pyruvate kinase	Phosphorylation	+ 2
	Consumption of ATP by reaction	Catalyzed by hexokinase and phosphofructokinase-I	− 2
		NET	2
	Lactate dehydrogenase	Respiratory chain	+ 6
	Pyruvate dehydrogenase	oxidation of 2NADH	+ 6
Citric acid cycle	Isocitrate dehydrogenase	Respiratory chain oxidation of 2NADH	6
	α-Ketoglutarate dehydrogenase	Respiratory chain oxidation of 2NADH	6
	Succinate thiokinase	Phosphorylation at substrate level	2
	Succinate dehydrogenase	Respiratory chain oxidation of 2FADH$_2$	4
	Malate dehydrogenase	Respiratory chain oxidation of 2NADH$_2$	6
		NET	36
	Total (Net) per mole of glucose under aerobic condition		36
	Total (Net) per mole of glucose under anerobic condition		2
	Grand total		38

cholesterol, steroid hormones, fatty acids and amino acids).

3. This pathway provides for the formation of pentoses for synthesis of nucleotides (RNA, DNA, CoA, NAD, FAD, ATP).

4. This pathway also provides for the synthesis of sugars with 3, 4, 5, 6, 7 carbon atoms.

5. Interconversion of various sugars is also possible in this pathway.

6. The activity of HMP is very low in skeletal muscle and very high in adipose tissue. It is active in liver, erythrocytes, testes, lactating mammary gland, adrenal cortex and thyroid.

The steps of pentose phosphate pathway are given in Fig. 7.10.

Uronic Acid Pathway

Apart from glycolysis, TCA cycle and HMP shunt pathway, another pathway for utilizing glucose also exists. This is known as uronic acid pathway.

The pathway is important as it forms glucuronic acid which is needed for synthesis of mucopolysaccharides like, chondroitin sulfate, and for conjugation of bilirubin, steroid hormones and certain drugs. In certain animals (monkeys, dogs and cats), ascorbic acid is synthesized from L-gulonic acid formed in this pathway. But in man and guinea pigs, the necessary enzymes for this conversion are lacking, hence, ascorbic acid is needed in their diet. The steps of this pathway are not described here.

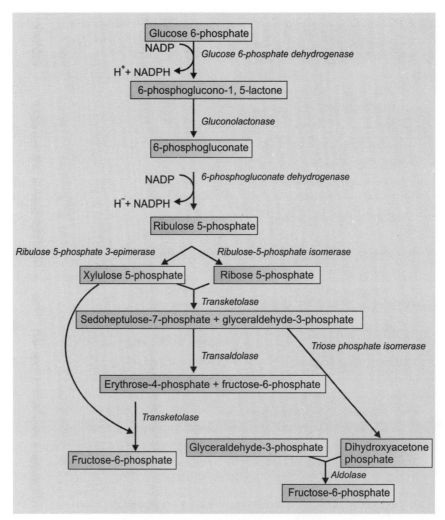

Fig. 7.10: Pentose phosphate pathway

GLUCONEOGENESIS

Apart from digestion, absorption and glycogen breakdown another process that contributes sugar to blood. Gluconeogenesis (or neoglucogenesis) means the synthesis of glucose from non-carbohydrate sources. It occurs mainly in liver and kidney. Lactate, glycerol and certain amino acids are major neoglucogenic substances.

Neoglucogenesis maintains the blood sugar level and meets body's need of glucose when diet is insufficient in carbohydrates or food absorption is over.

Gluconeogenesis is accomplished by reversal of glycolysis. Its metabolic pathway is shown in Fig. 7.11.

Most of the reactions of glycolysis are reversible. However, there are certain reactions which are irreversible on account of energy barriers (ATP hydrolysis). These are, therefore, bypassed by side reactions as shown below:

1. Glucose-6-phosphatase forms glucose from glucose-6-phosphate.
2. Fructose-1, 6-diphosphatase forms fructose-6-phosphate from fructose-1, 6-diphosphate.

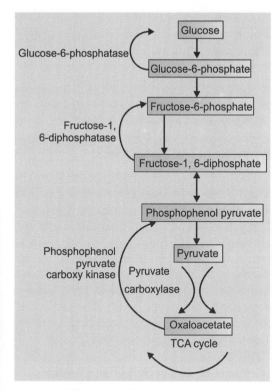

Fig. 7.11: Gluconeogenesis

3. Pyruvate carboxylase forms oxaloacetate from pyruvate.

4. Phosphoenol pyruvate carboxy kinase forms phosphoenol pyruvate from oxaloacetate in mitochondria. Since oxaloacetate is carrier molecule of TCA cycle, any intermediate of this cycle is capable of forming glucose by going in reverse.

With the help of these enzymes, any intermediate of glycolysis or TCA cycle can be used to form glucose. The neoglucogenesis is important in maintaining blood glucose when absorption is over. Three most important compounds in contributing glucose by neoglucogenesis are lactic acid, glycerol and amino acids.

Functions of Gluconeogenesis

1. During starvation or during periods of limited carbohydrate intake, when the level of liver glycogen is low, gluconeogenesis is important in maintaining blood glucose concentration.

2. Even when most of the energy requirement of the organism is met by the supply of fat, there is always a certain basal requirement of glucose which is provided by gluconeogenesis.

3. During extended exercise, when high catecholamine levels have mobilized carbohydrate and lipid reserves, the gluconeogenic pathway allows the use of lactate from glycolysis and glycerol from fat breakdown.

Substrates for Gluconeogenesis

Lactate: Lactate is the end product of glycolysis in skeletal muscles during anaerobic conditions. Its accumulation there can cause muscle fatigue, so it slowly diffuses into blood, enters liver where it is converted into glucose or glycogen. Glucose, so formed comes back into muscles through blood circulation for further glycolysis to continue. This is known as Cori's cycle. It functions to:

• Maintain glucose supply for vital tissues, and

• Prevent lactic acidosis due to an excess of lactate.

The steps involved:

The Cori's cycle

a. Pyruvate formed from glucose is converted to lactic acid by lactate dehydrogenase in the muscles cell.

b. Lactate is released into blood and taken up the liver.

c. Lactate is converted to pyruvate by the enzyme lactate dehydrogenase using NAD^+ as cofactor in the liver.

d. Pyruvate is converted to glucose by gluconeogenic mechanism in the liver and released into the blood where it can be used as an energy source for muscles and other tissues.

Pyruvate formed from glucose in the muscles can be converted to alanine as well.

Hence, alanine too can function as a substrate for gluconeogenesis, as we will discuss.

a. Pyruvate formed from glycolysis in the muscles is converted to alanine by transamination reaction.
b. Alanine released by the muscles is converted back to pyruvate by the reverse of transamination reaction that occurred in the muscles.
c. Pyruvate is converted to glucose via gluconeogenic pathway.
d. The NH_3 liberted is converted to urea in the liver.

Glycerol

Glycerol formed in adipose tissue is transported to liver for conversion into glucose or resynthesis of fat.

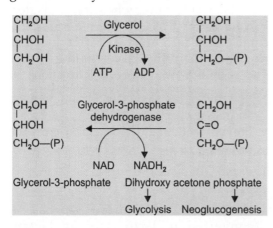

Glycerol-3-phosphate   Dihydroxy acetone phosphate

Amino Acids

Many amino acids are called glucogenic as their catabolism form one of the intermediate of glycolysis or citric acid cycle which can form glucose as shown above. The amino acids are classified in Table 7.3. According to the glycolytic intermediate, they form during their catabolism.

Two other processes removing glucose from blood are discussed below:

Synthesis of Fat (Lipogenesis)

Carbohydrates can easily form fat in the body. This is the reason why many people who do not consume much fat still get obese. The synthesis of fat requires fatty acid and glycerol. Acetyl coenzyme can be used to synthesize fatty acid in extra mitochondrial pathway. The glycerol moiety for combination with activated fatty acid is provided by glycolysis. The relevant compound is dihydroxyacetone phosphate (see above in neoglucogenesis).

Synthesis of Amino Acids and Proteins

Certain alpha keto acids (pyruvic acid, alpha keto glutaric acid, oxaloacetic acid) formed during catabolism of glucose yield corresponding amino acid on transamination, which may be used to form proteins.

BLOOD SUGAR AND ITS REGULATION

The body attempts to maintain the blood sugar (glucose) at a relatively constant level. The normal fasting (post-absorptive) venous blood sugar concentration averages about 80–120 mg/ml as determined by reduction

Table 7.3: Glucogenic amino acids				
Oxaloacetate	α-Ketoglutarate	Succinyl CoA	Fumarate	Pyruvate
Aspartate	Glutamate	Isoleucine	Tyrosine	Alanine
	Histidine	Methionine	Phenyl-	Tryptophan
	Proline	Valine	alanine	Methionine
	Hydroxyproline		Threonine	Serine, cysteine
	Arginine			

methods. However, true sugar values are (60–100 mg%) estimated by enzyme method. The blood sugar level reflects equilibrium between factors supplying sugar to the blood and those removing it from the blood (Fig. 7.12). Arterial blood contains 2–10 mg% more than venous blood. After meals, blood sugar rises to 120–130 mg% and after fast drops to 60–70 mg%. The regulation of sugar level in blood is mainly accomplished by hormones.

Hormonal Regulation of Blood Sugar

A number of hormones are there which either add or remove glucose in blood (Fig. 7.12). How hormones act on organs is shown in Fig. 7.13.

Hormones Decreasing Blood Sugar Level

Insulin: This hormone is secreted by β-cells of pancreas. It decreases blood sugar level by favoring glycogenesis in liver and increased use of glucose in other tissues. It increases permeability for glucose in peripheral tissues by inducing hexokinase. Secretion of insulin increases in response to rise in blood sugar level and *vice versa*.

Hormones Increasing Blood Sugar Level

1. **Adrenaline or epinephrine:** It is secreted by adrenal medulla. It acts opposite to that of insulin. It favors glycogenolysis in liver and muscle by stimulating phosphorylase and it appears to decrease uptake of glucose by tissue cells. It is secreted in stress, anxiety, fear, etc.

2. **Glucagon:** It is secreted by α-cells of pancreas. It stimulates glycogenolysis in liver by the similar mechanism.

3. **Glucocorticoids:** These hormones are secreted by adrenal cortex. These stimulate gluconeogenesis by increasing protein catabolism. It inhibits utilization of glucose in extra hepatic tissues. Thus, all the actions of glucocorticoids are antagonistic to insulin.

4. **Thyroid hormone:** It is secreted by thyroid gland. It should also be considered as hormone affecting the blood sugar level. It stimulates hepatic glycogenolysis. It also affects the intestinal absorption of sugar.

5. **Anterior pituitary hormone:** Adreno-corticotropic (ACTH) and Thyrotropic (TSH) hormones generally produce the same effects as glucocorticoids and thyroxine because of their actions in stimulating the production of latter hormones. Other factors from the anterior pituitary also have hyperglycemic activity. Growth hormone decrease glucose uptake in muscle, increases

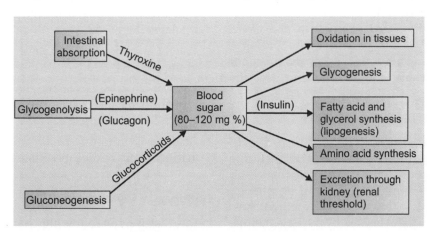

Fig. 7.12: Blood sugar regulation

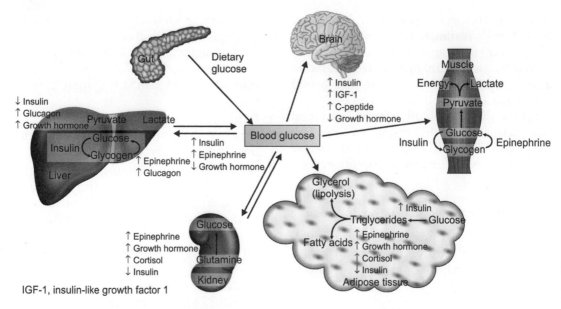

Fig. 7.13: Schematic overview of hormonal control of blood glucose

glucose by sparing action (fat mobilization). Thus, ultimate control of blood sugar concentration depends on a delicate balance between the various hormones.

Renal Control

Kidney plays an important role in control of blood sugar. Glucose is filtered in glomerulus and is reabsorbed in renal tubules. The reabsorption is a rate limiting factor. If the blood sugar level is raised above 180 mg/100 ml, complete tubular reabsorption of sugar does not occur and the extra amount appears in the urine causing glucosuria. This level is known as renal threshold value.

DIABETES MELLITUS

Diabetes mellitus is a condition due to absolute or relative lack of the hormone insulin resulting in primary disturbances in carbohydrate metabolism and secondary disturbances in fat and protein metabolisms. Diabetes is characterized by hyperglycemia, glycosuria, polyuria, ketosis, acidosis, etc.

Symptoms

- *Hyperglycemia (high blood sugar):* Due to poor control, blood sugar is raised above the normal value.

- *Glycosuria (glucose in urine):* Once renal threshold is crossed, glucose spills into urine.

- *Polyuria (increased urine output):* In order to remove glucose in solution, more urine is passed.

- *Polydipsia (excessive thrust):* To compensate excessive micturition, water intake is increased.

- *Weight loss:* Because nutrient glucose is going as waste.

- *Ketosis:* Glucose is wasted, so energy is supplied by excessive fat catabolism which leads to ketosis.

- *Acidosis:* Occurs due to accumulation of acidic ketone bodies in ketosis.

Changes in Metabolism

In this disease, the following changes occur in the metabolism.

1. Carbohydrate Metabolism

- Glycogen content decreases in liver as more and more glycogen is converted to glucose.
- Hyperglycemia, i.e. increased blood glucose level.
- Glycosuria: Excess of glucose is given out in urine.

2. Fat Metabolism

- Fat synthesis decreases.
- Ketosis occurs in long run.
- Acidosis occurs in long run.

3. Protein Metabolism

- Protein metabolism increases.
- Gluconeogenesis increases, i.e. more and more of amino acids are converted to glucose.

Laboratory Diagnosis

- Blood glucose estimation. Fasting and 2 hours post meal (postprandial) samples
- Glucose tolerance test (GTT)
- Blood glycosylated hemoglobin test (HbA$_{1C}$)
- Blood lipid profile test
- Urine glucose and ketone test.

GLUCOSE TOLERANCE TEST (GTT)

Glucose tolerance is ability to utilize carbohydrates. It is indicated by the nature of blood glucose curve following the administration of glucose. The 'glucose tolerance' is a valuable diagnostic aid (Fig. 7.14).

Procedure

1. After an overnight (12 hours) fasting, blood sample is collected.
2. The bladder is emptied completely and urine is collected for qualitative test for glucose and ketone bodies. This is fasting urine sample.
3. About 50 to 75 grams of glucose powder dissolved in 250 ml of water is given to the individual to drink. Time of oral glucose administration is noted.
4. Five specimen samples of venous blood and urine are collected every 30 minutes after the oral glucose viz. 30 min, 60 min, 90 min, 120 min and 150 minutes.
5. Glucose content of all the blood samples are estimated and plotted graphically. The nature of curve gives an idea of glucose utilization.

GLYCEMIC INDEX

Carbohydrates are universal constituents of most of the food stuffs. They are an

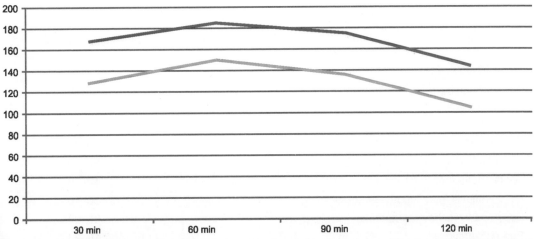

Fig. 7.14: Normal glucose tolerance curve (light colored) and abnormal glucose tolerance curve (dark colored)

indispensable part of a healthy diet. The carbohydrates after digestion releaseses monosaccharides which in the body are converted into glucose. The effect of different foods on raising blood glucose level varies considerably. The glycemic index provides a mathematical expression of the extent of rise in blood glucose level following consumption of a particular food item, in comparison to rise in blood glucose relative to consumption of pure glucose. The glycemic index of glucose is taken as 100.

Glycemic index is calculated from the curves obtained in glucose tolerance test. The area under the two hour plasma glucose curve after eating food (test meal) is compared to the area under the blood glucose curve after eating the same amount of pure glucose (usually 50 grams). It is expressed as percentage.

$$\text{Glycemic index} = \frac{\text{Area under blood glucose curve after ingestion of meal}}{\text{Area under the curve after ingestion of glucose}} \times 100$$

Foods are ranked based on how they compare to reference food, i.e. glucose. Foods with a glycemic index of 55 or less are classified as low glycemic index, those which score between 56 and 69 are medium glycemic index and those which score 70 and above, have a high glycemic index.

High glycemic index foods cause a sharp spike in blood glucose level. Foods with a low glycemic index have a slower and steadier effect on blood sugar.

The glycemic index of carbohydrates is lowered if it is combined with fiber, proteins or lipids. Ice cream though contains high sugar but it has a low glycemic index because it contains lot of fat which prevents rapid glucose absorption.

The glycemic index is useful in formulating diets for diabetic persons. It gives information about which food is good for people with diabetes. Large amount of low glycemic index foods are included in diabetic diet because it prevents rapid rise in blood sugar and helps in managing blood glucose level. Sugars, sweets and refined carbohydrates should be avoided because high glycemic index foods are associated with increased risk of obesity, diabetes mellitus and cardiovascular diseases.

GLYCOSURIA

It is a condition in which sugar is present in urine. In most of the cases, the sugar is glucose. It occurs due to the following causes:

i. **Alimentary:** When excess of carbohydrate is present in food, it sometimes spills in urine. It is transitory.

Table 7.4: Glycemic index of some common food stuffs

Food items	Glycemic index (glucose = 100)
White rice/rice cakes	90–95
Table sugar/sparkling glucose drinks	85–90
Cornflakes/potato/honey	80–85
Bread/wafers/watermelon/pizza/soft drinks	70–80
Banana/raisins/grains/cookies	60–70
Oat meal/sweet corn/grapes	50–60
Apple/orange/peach/cakes	40–50
Ice cream/milk/pear/legumes/carrots	30–40
Soya beans/cashews/vegetables	20–30
Pea nuts/fructose	10–20

ii. Renal: Due to the defect in renal tubules, the renal threshold is lowered so sugar appears in urine though the blood sugar level remains normal.

iii. Diabetic: It occurs due to insulin deficiency. The renal threshold is normal; sugar appears in urine when it is crossed.

In some rare cases, sugars other than glucose may appear in urine which may give positive reducing test. These are listed further.

Substances giving a positive reducing test in urine are:

Glucose: In diabetes mellitus.

Lactose: During lactation and last trimester of pregnancy.

Galactose: In galactosemia and galactokinase deficiency.

Fructose: In hereditary fructose intolerance and essential fructosuria.

Pentoses: After eating certain fruits and in essential pentosuria.

Homogentisic acid: In alkaptonuria.

Glucuronides of certain drugs: On ingestion of certain drugs.

Salicylic acid: In aspirin overdose.

Ascorbic acid: With high vitamin C intake.

Creatinine: Only in high concentration.

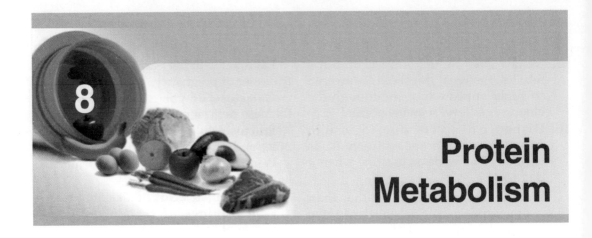

Protein
Metabolism

INTRODUCTION

Proteins are molecules formed by the combination of a number of L-alpha amino acids. Natural human proteins are made up of only 20 α-amino acids, all of which belong to L-type. Each amino acid combines with other amino acid by a reaction between amino groups of one amino acid to carboxyl group of another amino acid. A molecule of water is driven out and the two amino acids are united by a specific peptide (CO–NH) linkage. This reaction can be repeated using same or different amino acids. The amino acid chain is thus lengthened gradually in linear fashion. By using different amino acids or repeating others, innumerable different proteins are produced, which differ in their sequence of amino acids. The long chain of amino acids then acquires compact globular shape by folding of the molecule by means of hydrogen bonds and other non-covalent forces.

When food is eaten, its constituents undergo various transformations in the body. This is known as *metabolism*. It is of two types—*anabolism* and *catabolism*. The anabolism is synthesis of large molecule from smaller ones, while catabolism means breakdown of big molecules into simpler units. Generally, anabolism requires consumption of energy to accomplish the reaction. On the other hand, catabolic reactions are mostly accompanied by liberation of energy. All these chemical reactions occur inside the cell. These reactions are preceded by *digestion* and *absorption* of food constituents. The food is mostly cooked before eating because the ingredients of food in its native state are very difficult to digest.

EFFECT OF COOKING

The cooking includes the application of heat in some or the other form—boiling, frying, stewing or steaming. Cooking makes food more easily digestible.

Heat denatures nature of proteins. It involves the unfolding of folded protein molecule which exposes many hidden peptide bonds for the action of enzymes. This proteolytic denaturation is also aided by the gastric HCl when food comes in the stomach.

METABOLISM

An overview of the complete metabolism of proteins in the body is given in Fig. 8.1.

Now we discuss different aspects of protein metabolism.

Digestion

The digestion and absorption occur in the gastrointestinal tract. The aim of digestion

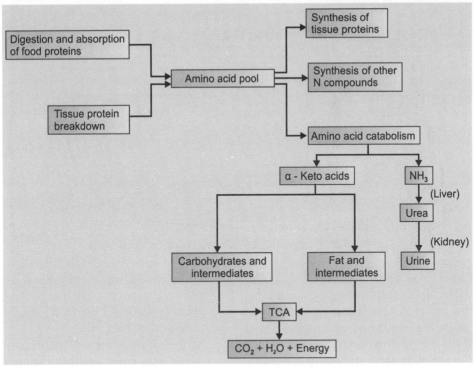

Fig. 8.1: Overview of protein metabolism

is to convert complex, high molecular weight, colloidal and insoluble substances into simple, soluble, low molecular weight substances which are easily absorbed. Protein digestion starts in the stomach and is completed in small intestine (Fig. 8.2).

The digestion of proteins is carried out by proteolytic (protein splitting) enzymes in the gut. Proteolytic enzymes are generally secreted in the inactive form called *zymogens*. HCl or another enzyme converts them into active enzyme. The protein is first acted upon by such enzymes which convert them into several polypeptide fragments (endopeptidases). Later on these polypeptide fragments are acted upon by a set of enzymes which convert them into individual amino acids (exopeptidases). The different proteolytic enzymes acting on protein molecule in the gut are discussed below.

Stomach: *Pepsin* is the first proteolytic enzyme to act. It acts on peptide bonds formed by acidic amino acids.

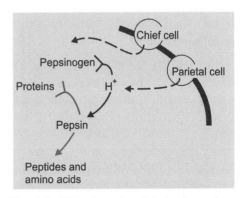

Fig. 8.2: Digestion of protein in stomach

Pancreatic juice: It contains many proteolytic enzymes. *Trypsin* cleaves peptide bonds involving basic amino acids. *Chymotrypsin* hydrolyses peptide bonds formed by aromatic amino acids. *Carboxypeptidase* breaks peptide bond near a free carboxylic group. By this stage, the protein is fragmented into smaller peptides (Fig. 8.3).

Intestinal Juice: It contains a number of peptidase. *Amino peptidase* acts on peptide

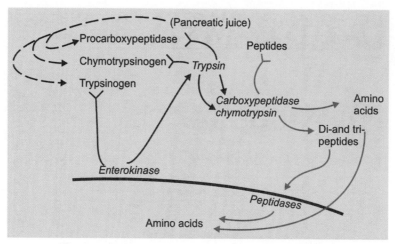

Fig. 8.3: Pancreatic and intestinal digestion of proteins

bond near free amino group, while tri-peptidase and dipeptidase act on tripeptides and dipeptides to give free amino acids.

Thus, by the combined action of all these enzymes, 90–95% of food proteins are completely digested into amino acids, which are absorbed. Undigested protein is passed into feces.

Absorption

As amino acids are water soluble, their absorption occurs by portal venous system. The mechanism of absorption (Fig. 8.4) is similar to the mechanism of absorption of glucose. The salient features of absorption are described below:

1. All amino acids (both L- and D-types) are capable of absorption by passive diffusion, but L-amino acids are mainly absorbed by the active process.

2. The absorption occurs by jejunum and ileum.

3. The absorption is very rapid and complete; as much as 95% of liberated amino acids are absorbed.

4. The amino N level in blood in fasting conditions is 4–6 mg/100 ml which rises by 2–4 mg/100 ml after absorption from meals.

5. The absorption is carrier-mediated active process, requiring energy by hydrolysis of ATP and B_6-PO_4 and co-transport of Na^+ ion.

6. All 20 amino acids are not absorbed at a single site. There are four different sites for absorption—for basic amino acids, acidic amino acids, neutral amino acids and imino acids.

7. A specific transport protein at these sites on the cell membranes binds a particular amino acid and Na^+ ion from the intestinal lumen.

8. The carrier protein delivers both the sodium ion and amino acid into cytosol of intestinal cell and itself comes back to ferry another molecule of amino acid.

9. From the cytosol, the amino acid goes to portal circulation, while the sodium ion is pumped back into the lumen by the energy derived from ATP hydrolysis by an enzyme called Na^+-K^+-ATPase, which simultaneously propels potassium ion (K^+) from lumen into the intestinal cell.

10. Small amount of di- and tri-peptides may be absorbed, which are digested by intracellular di- and tri-peptidases.

11. In newborn infants, immunoglobulins (gamma globulins) present in the mother's milk (colostrum) secreted

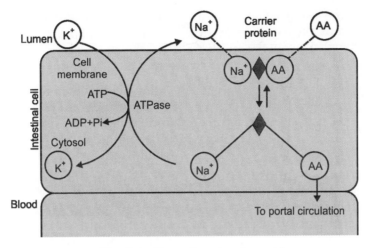

Fig. 8.4: Absorption of amino acids

during initial few days impart passive immunity to the child.

12. Sometimes, some adults absorb whole protein molecule by endocytosis which acts as antigen which excite immunologic reactions or allergic reaction. This is the cause of food allergy observed in some people.

AMINO ACID POOL

The central theme in the outline of protein metabolism is existence of an 'amino acid pool'. It is the presence of the amino acid in the blood. These are contributed by processes shown in Fig. 8.1. These are:

1. Digestion and absorption of dietary protein
2. Tissue protein breakdown.

Amino acids derived from these two processes mix and become indistinguishable. Amino acids of the pool account for about 2 g nitrogen. These amino acids are utilized in the processes as shown in Fig. 8.1, viz.

1. Amino acid catabolism
2. Synthesis of tissue proteins
3. Synthesis of other nitrogenous compounds.

Processes which Contribute Amino Acids to the Pool

1. Digestion and absorption of dietary protein: Already discussed in the beginning.
2. Tissue protein breakdown: Human tissues are made up of proteins. The tissues are not static deposits of proteins. Rather the tissue protein molecules are constantly being broken down and rebuilt. Thus, an individual having constant weight is in equilibrium with respect to degradation and rebuilding of his tissues. Such an individual is said to be in nitrogen equilibrium and the constituents are referred as having *dynamic state of body constituents*. The rate at which a tissue regenerates its proteins differ considerably, this is called *protein turnover*. This is expressed in terms of 'half life'. The 'half life' is the number of days within which a tissue regenerates half of its proteins. This differs considerably for different tissues. The protein turnover is greatest in intestinal mucosa followed by kidney, liver, brain and muscle in that order.

Nitrogen Balance

The only source of nitrogen to the body is food proteins. The body loses nitrogen mainly in the urine (as urea, uric acid, creatinine, etc.) and partly in feces (as unabsorbed proteins). This intake and loss from the body can be analyzed. If the intake of nitrogen of a person equals losses, the person is said to be in nitrogen equilibrium or nitrogen balance. This occurs in healthy adults who maintain constant weight. If the nitrogen intake exceeds the losses, the person is said to be in positive nitrogen balance. This occurs in children during growth. Sometimes, the intake is less than the losses, then the person is said to be in negative nitrogen balance. This occurs in wasting diseases and fever.

Nitrogen balance
    N intake = N output
Positive nitrogen balance
    N intake > N output
Negative nitrogen balance
    N intake < N output

Processes which Remove Amino Acids from the Pool

The processes shown in Fig. 8.1 are those which remove amino acids from amino acid pool. The major portion of amino acids is utilized in the synthesis of proteins of tissues. This is the primary function of dietary proteins. Apart from it, all nitrogenous substances in the body are ultimately synthesized from amino acids. The amino acids not utilized in above processes are degraded. This is called amino acid catabolism. The catabolic process is responsible for two important functions:

1. Release of energy to the body and
2. Formation of urea for excretion in urine.

We will first discuss catabolism of amino acids in this chapter and then anabolism.

AMINO ACID CATABOLISM

Amino acid catabolism can be conveniently discussed in three parts:

a. Removal of ammonia

b. Utilization of ammonia
c. Utilization of α-keto acids.

Removal of Ammonia

Amino acids which are not used for synthesis are catabolized by various reactions, predominantly in liver. The various reactions which occur are transamination, deamination, oxidative deamination, etc.

i. Transamination: In transamination, an amino acid reacts with a keto acid to exchange amino group and keto group between them. This produces keto acid corresponding to amino acid and amino acid corresponding to keto acid.

R_1	R_2		R_1	R_2
$\mid$	$\mid$		$\mid$	$\mid$
$CH\ NH_3^+$ +	$C=O$		$C=O$ +	$CH\ NH_3$
$\mid$	$\mid$		$\mid$	$\mid$
COO^-	COO^-		COO^-	COO^-
Amino acid (R1)	Keto acid (R2)		Keto acid (R1)	Amino acid (R2)

α-ketoglutarate plays a significant role in amino acid metabolism by accepting the amino groups from other amino acids, thus, forming glutamate. The reaction of transamination is catalyzed by aminotransferase (transaminase). The two most important transferases are:

a. Alanine aminotransferase (ALT/SGPT)

Alanine + α-ketoglutarate ⟷
Glutamate + Pyruvate

b. Aspartate aminotransferase (AST/SGOT)

Asparate + α-ketoglutarate ⟷
Oxaloacetate + Glutamate
(OR)

Glutamate + Pyruvate $\xleftrightarrow{GPT}$ α-ketoglutarate + Alanine

Glutamate + Oxaloacetate $\xleftrightarrow{GOT}$ α-ketoglutarate + Aspartate

It may be noted that:
1. Puruvate, oxaloacetate and α-ketoglutarate are intermediates of glucose breakdown.

2. This reaction makes it possible to synthesize non-essential amino acids.

3. The enzymes which catalyze these reactions are called transaminases —GPT is glutamate pyruvate transaminase and GOT is glutamate oxaloacetate transaminase.

4. These transaminases contain pyridoxal phosphate (B_6-PO_4) as the coenzyme part, and

5. Transaminases level in blood is estimated to diagnose certain diseases of heart and liver.

Transamination using glutamine and asparagine (which are amides of glutamate and aspartate, respectively) is more rapid, extensive and important in liver. There is exchange of amino group and α-keto group with removal of amide group as ammonia.

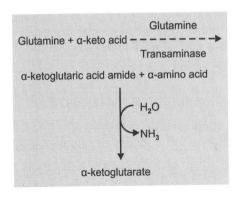

This reaction is catalyzed by glutamine transaminase which is also having pyridoxal phosphate (B_6-PO_4) as coenzyme.

ii. Oxidative deamination: A major part of ammonia is liberated from amino acids by reaction known as oxidative deamination, which means oxidation (removal of hydrogen) coupled to removal of ammonia. There are two enzymes for these types of reactions.

a. *Glutamate dehydrogenase:* It catalyzes the deamination of most of the amino acids in many tissues. The reaction is essentially transamination followed by deamination.

α-amino acid + α-ketoglutarate

Transaminase ↓

α-keto acid + Glutamate

Glutamate dehydrogenase ↓ +H_2O + NAD

α-ketoglutarate + $NADH_2$ + NH_3

b. *Amino acid oxidase:* This enzyme can also oxidize amino acids directly to form α-keto acids liberating free ammonia.

$$L\text{-amino acid} \xrightarrow[\text{A.A. oxidase}]{+H_2O + FMN} \alpha\text{-keto acid} + NH_3 + FMNH_2$$

Utilization of Ammonia

Ammonia produced by these reactions is very toxic especially to the brain and central nervous system. Therefore, it needs to be immediately converted into urea which is a neutral compound. This occurs in liver. The overall reaction is:

$$2NH_3 + CO_2 \rightarrow NH_2CONH_2 + H_2O$$

But it does not form directly as shown above, but sequentially by a series of reactions.

Urea Formation

The synthesis of urea in liver occurs by a closed sequence of reactions known as urea cycle or Krebs-Hensleit cycle. In this cycle, several amino acids take part and ornithine acts as a carrier molecule. The first two reactions occur in the mitochondria and rest in the cytosol.

These reactions are described further. The amino group of all amino acids is ultimately converted to ammonia (NH_3). Ammonia is highly toxic to the nervous system. Hence, it must be removed immediately. So ammonia combines with CO_2 to form urea, which is not toxic to the body. Hence, one of the major end products of protein metabolism is urea. Urea is produced by the liver and is then transported in the blood to the kidneys for excretion in the urine. The steps involved in converting ammonia to urea includes:

1. Formation of carbamoyl phosphate. This occurs in two steps. The enzyme is a synthetase (carbamoyl phosphate synthetase).

$$CO_2 \xrightarrow{\quad\quad} \text{Active "}CO_2\text{"}$$
$$ATP \quad ADP + Pi$$

$$\text{Active "}CO_2\text{"} + NH_3 \xrightarrow{\quad\quad} \text{Carbamoyl phosphate}$$
$$ATP \quad ADP$$

Carbamoyl group is, $NH_2.CO$; thus two-thirds of urea molecule is synthesized in first reaction. The remaining reactions are meant to add another NH_2 group.

2. Transfer of carbamoyl group to ornithine. The reaction is catalyzed by a transferase, called ornithine transcarbamoylase.

$$\text{Ornithine + Carbamoyl phosphate} \xrightarrow{Pi} \text{Citrulline}$$

Citrulline formed leaves mitochondria and enter cytosol to undergo further reactions.

3. Condensation of citrulline with aspartate catalyzed by a condensing enzyme arginosuccinate synthase.

Citrulline + Asparate + ATP → Argininosuccinate
$+H_2O$ +AMP + PPi

4. Breakdown of argininosuccinate by the enzyme argininosuccinase.

Argininosuccinate → Arginine + Fumarate

Fumarate goes to mitochondria and is converted there into oxaloacetate in TCA cycle. Oxaloacetate comes back in cytoplasm and is converted into aspartic acid by transamination, which is needed in reaction number 3. Thus, urea cycle is integrated to TCA cycle.

5. Formation of urea by splitting arginine by enzyme arginase.

Arginine + H_2O → Ornithine + Urea

Thus, ornithine is regenerated at the end of the cycle to restart another round of urea cycle.

Notes:

- It may be noted that urea synthesis occurs at the expense of four high energy phosphate bonds of ATP.
- In liver diseases, urea synthesis is impaired, so ammonia accumulates in the blood which causes coma and ultimately death. Ammonia accumulation (hyperammonemia) affects speech and vision and causes tremors.

Utilization of α-Keto Acids

The removal of ammonia from the amino acids produces α-keto acids. These are intermediates of TCA cycle or glycolysis. The reversal of this pathway synthesizes glucose (neoglucogenesis). Such amino acids are called glycogenic amino acids, and this is how proteins are converted into carbohydrates for giving energy by oxidation. A few amino acids (leucine and isoleucine) on degradation form ketone bodies, viz. instead of carbohydrates. These are referred to as ketogenic amino acids.

SYNTHESIS OF TISSUE PROTEINS

The main function of dietary proteins is to synthesize new tissues or replace old worn out tissues. About 400 g protein is formed and degraded everyday in an adult person. The protein synthesis is very complicated process. We shall present here a very simplified version. For its understanding, you should have a clear idea of chemistry of nucleic acids (Chapter 11) and amino acids (Chapter 2).

Site

Protein synthesis takes place on rough endoplasmic reticulum. The ribosomes act as "work benches" or factories for synthesis of proteins.

Components

The various components required for protein synthesis are—DNA, RNA (mRNA, t-RNA), ribosomes and amino acids. The 20 amino acids are described in Chapter 2.

i. DNA

It is present in the nucleus. It has two strands of nucleotides which are complementary to each other. Each strand contains about 1 million (1×10^6) nucleotides. It contains the information or "Blueprint" about the proteins to be synthesized. This information is coded in the form of sequence of nucleotides or bases. DNA forms different RNAs by transcription.

ii. RNA

Three types of RNA are required for protein synthesis. All these are formed from DNA.

a. **mRNA:** Messenger RNA (mRNA) acts as a 'template' or mould for protein synthesis. It is single stranded molecule containing about 3000 nucleotides.

b. **tRNA:** The transfer RNA (tRNA), also called soluble RNA (sRNA) is short chain of about 73–93 nucleotides folded in a 'clover leaf' structure. Their function is to carry amino acids. There are different tRNAs for different amino acids. The specificity for amino acid lies in the three base pairs called 'anticodon'. The amino acid binds to 3′ end which has C-C-AOH (cytidylic acid-cytidylic acid-adenosine).

c. **rRNA:** A ribosome contains a number of proteins and various RNA molecules which are called ribosomal RNA (rRNA).

iii. Ribosomes

Ribosomes are spherical particles which can be dissociated into two parts—small subunit and large subunit. The small subunit contains site for binding to mRNA and also has mechanism for moving mRNA by three nucleotides. The large subunit has two sites for binding tRNAs. It also contains the enzyme peptidyl transferase which establishes peptide bond between existing peptide chain and incoming amino acid.

iv. Amino Acids

Last but not the least, all the 20 L-α amino acids are required to synthesize proteins.

GENETIC CODE

DNA and RNA are polynucleotides in which only bases vary. Out of four bases present in DNA—adenine (A), guanine (G), cytosine (C) and thymine (T), three consecutive bases signify one amino acid. This relationship is called genetic code.

The genetic code (Table 8.1) is the basis of heredity. For triplet code 4^3(64), different combinations are possible. Since these combinations, called codes, are to denote only 20 amino acids, multiple codes exist for one amino acid. Apart from this, some code words signify protein chain initiation (beginning) and some termination (end of synthesis). The four bases can be likened to 'letters' in a language and triplet code to the 'words'. The information coded in base sequence of DNA is first fully transferred to mRNA whose bases are same except uracil replaces thymine. The message in mRNA is contained as a continuous sequence of bases without coma or full stop or overlapping. It is read sequentially, for example,

AUGGCGUUCGUACUUAAA-UAUGGAAUC............

The genetic code is universal, that means it remains same in all forms of life. **It is the language of life.** The meaning of all 64 possible combinations has been deciphered by scientists and it is now well known. It is generally shown in the tabular form and called the 'genetic code' (Table 8.1).

Processes

Protein synthesis basically involves two major processes—transcription and translation.

Table 8.1: The genetic code

1st letter	2nd letter				3rd letter
	U	C	A	G	
U	PHE	SER	TYR	CYS	U
	PHE	SER	TYR	CYS	C
	LEU	SER	CT	CT	A
	LEU	SER	CT	TRY	G
C	LEU	PRO	HIS	ARG	U
	LEU	PRO	HIS	ARG	C
	LEU	PRO	GLN	ARG	A
	LEU	PRO	GLN	ARG	G
A	ILEU	THR	ASN	SER	U
	ILEU	THR	ASN	SER	C
	ILEU	THR	LYS	ARG	A
	MET; CI	THR	LYS	ARG	G
G	VAL	ALA	ASP	GLY	U
	VAL	ALA	ASP	GLY	C
	VAL	ALA	GLU	GLY	A
	VAL; CI	ALA	GLU	GLY	G

Note: U: uracil; C: cytosine; A: adenine; G: guanine
CI: chain initiation; CT: chain termination
Amino acids are represented by their usual abbreviations.

Transcription

It is actually the synthesis of mRNA from DNA. As in literature, transcription means change of script of one language into the script of another language. For example, "YOU GO" in English script becomes 'यू गो' in Hindi script. Similarly, the script of DNA (containing A, T, G, C) is converted into script of mRNA (containing U, A, C, G). Thus, in this process, transmission of genetic information occurs from nuclear DNA to cytoplasmic protein synthesizing sites by forming mRNA. The reaction is catalyzed by the enzyme RNA polymerase and takes place using intermediate formation of hybrid helix.

Translation

Translation in protein synthesis is the synthesis of protein as directed by information in mRNA. In the literature, translation means conversion of message of one language into another language. Thus, the message "YOU GO" in English when translated into Hindi will become 'तुम जाओ'. In protein synthesis, the language of mRNA (triplet codons of bases) is converted or translated into language of proteins (sequence of amino acids).

The amino acids do not directly recognize particular regions of mRNA. Instead, an adaptor molecule (tRNA) is involved which binds to particular region of mRNA codon by hydrogen bonding between complementary bases present in anticodon of tRNA. mRNA is decoded from the 5′, end towards the 3′, end and codons read in this order correspond to amino acids beginning from N-terminal and proceeding towards C-terminal end of the protein synthesized (Fig. 8.5).

Steps

There are three chemical steps in the synthesis of proteins.

1. **Activation of amino acids:** First, the amino acids are activated by the specific enzymes using energy from hydrolysis of ATP.

$$AA + ATP + E \longrightarrow E\text{-}AMP\text{-}AA$$

Amino acid   Activated amino acid

Enzyme (E)—specific amino acid activating enzyme

In this process, two high energy bonds are used.

2. **Transfer of amino acid to tRNA:** The amino acids are then transferred to respective tRNAs.

$$E\text{-}AMP\text{-}AA + tRNA \longrightarrow tRNA\text{-}AA \longrightarrow AMP + E$$

The enzyme is a transferase.

3. **Transfer of tRNA-AA to mRNA:** Amino acids come on mRNA one-by-one in accordance with codons on it. GTP supplies necessary energy. Amino acids thus join to form peptide bonds. The tRNAs are released to bring another molecule of same amino acid. All this reaction is catalyzed by the enzyme peptidyl transferase.

$$AA_1\text{-}tRNA_1 + AA_2\text{-}tRNA_2$$

$$+\ GTP \downarrow Peptidyl\ transferase$$

$$AA_1\text{-}AA_2\text{-}tRNA_2 + tRNA_1$$

Thus, three high energy bonds are consumed in forming one peptide bond.

The above cycle continues till whole proteins molecule is synthesized.

Mechanism

The mechanism of protein synthesis is as follows:

1. **Chain initiation:** The protein chain synthesis begins at the site on mRNA, where the chain initiation codon is present, i.e. AUG or GUG.

2. **Chain elongation:** Once started, protein chain synthesis proceeds rapidly as described above. Each ribosome is capable of incorporating 10 to 20 amino acids per second. On an average, there are 20,000 ribosomes in a cell, so 2 to 4 lacs of amino acids can combine in a second. Hence, the protein synthesis takes place very rapidly.

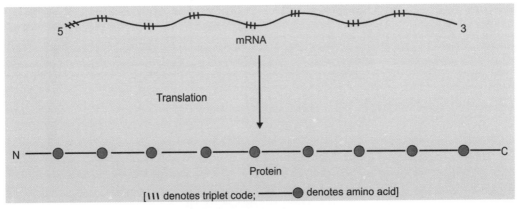

[\\\ denotes triplet code; —● denotes amino acid]

Fig. 8.5: Process of translation

3. Chain termination: The synthesis of protein chain stops on encountering chain termination codons. These are UAA, UAG and UGA.

SYNTHESIS OF OTHER NITROGENOUS COMPOUNDS

The amino acids also serve to synthesize all other nitrogen containing compounds in the body because nitrogen is contained only in proteins and not the carbohydrates or fat of the diet. Some important nitrogen containing compounds synthesized are— purines and pyrimidines (for nucleic acids), porphyrins (for heme compounds), glutathione, bile salts, urea, uric acid, creatine and creatinine.

Inhibitors of Protein Synthesis

Some substances inhibit process of protein synthesis at some or the other step. These are used as antibiotics. Antibiotics inhibit bacterial protein synthesis and thus kill the bacteria. Some examples are: Tetracycline, Chloramphenicol, Erythromycin, Streptomycin, Gentamycin. Others are Actinomycin D, Rifampin and Pyromycin.

Mutation

Mutation is the change in a single base of the nucleotide sequence of DNA genome. This change will pass on to mRNA and will result into the synthesis of a protein differing in the amino acid corresponding to the altered code.

The mutation is of two types:

1. Point Mutation

In point mutation, a single base is altered, so the resulting protein is different from normal protein in one amino acid only. Many hereditary diseases are due to it, e.g. different hemoglobins.

2. Frame Shift Mutation

It occurs by deletion or insertion of a base with the result that whole reading frame is altered, which may produce totally different protein. A mutation may be caused by X-rays, ionizing radiations, cosmic rays, certain chemicals, pollutants and atomic explosions which release enormous radiations. This is the real danger of atomic war or atomic explosions. The pregnancy of a woman in old age on account of late marriage or otherwise, carries a greater danger of having a malformed fetus (teratogenesis) because ova are already stored in the ovary. With increasing age, there is greater danger of mutation in nuclear DNA of the ovum. On the other hand, sperms in a man are formed fresh regularly in a short period and soon destroyed with less chances of being affected by mutation.

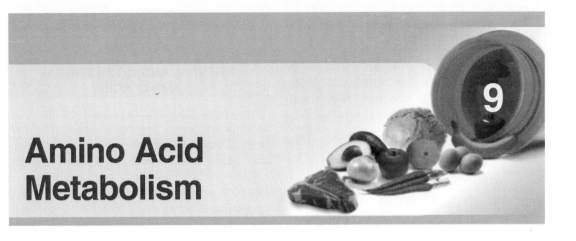

Amino Acid Metabolism

INTRODUCTION

The nitrogen enters the body through a variety of compounds present in the food, the most important being amino acids present in dietary proteins. The primary role of amino acids is in the synthesis of tissue protein and biosynthetic reactions. However, amino acids which cannot be used for biosynthesis are degraded. This scheme of things involves the following reactions (Fig. 9.1).

• The removal of α-amino groups (amino groups attached to carbon atom next to the carboxyl carbon) by two processes called transamination and oxidative deamination, forming ammonia and corresponding α-keto acids.

• The conversion of ammonia to urea in the urea cycle. A portion of the free ammonia is also excreted in urine as ammonium salt.

• Urea is the excretory end product of amino acid metabolism

The amino acids that are released by the hydrolysis of dietary and tissue protein mix with other amino acids distributed throughout the body. This is called amino acid pool. As you know there are 20 L-α amino acids in the proteins present in the

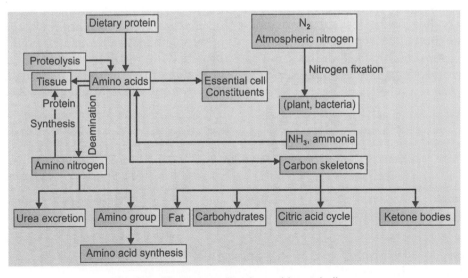

Fig. 9.1: Nitrogen and amino acid metabolism

body. It is not possible to discuss the metabolism of so many individual amino acids. Hence, certain common features of amino acid synthesis and breakdown will be discussed.

SYNTHESIS OF AMINO ACIDS

The routes of synthesis and of degradation are similar for some amino acids but not for others. Most amino acids arise from one of the five starting compounds: glutamate, oxaloacetate, pyruvate, phosphoenol pyruvate or glycerate-3-phosphate (Table 9.1).

Breakdown of Amino Acids

The amino acids are broadly considered as glucogenic or ketogenic or both glucogenic and ketogenic on the basis of their end product, being capable of forming glucose or ketone bodies, respectively. However, the amino acids have been grouped into five families on the basis of their final degradation products (Table. 9.2).

Pyruvate and Kreb's cycle intermediates can be converted to glucose, hence, first four groups of amino acids are known as 'glucogenic'. Acetyl CoA and acetoacetyl CoA cannot give rise to glucose, but form ketone bodies; hence, last group of amino acids are termed as 'ketogenic'.

The relationship of amino acid to carbohydrates and ketone bodies is shown in Fig. 9.2.

ESSENTIAL AND NON-ESSENTIAL AMINO ACIDS

The amino acids can be classified into two categories depending on whether they can be synthesized in the body. Many organisms including most plants and many micro-organisms, are capable of synthesizing all of the 20 amino acids that are normal constituents of proteins. In other organisms, particularly higher animals, the ability to synthesize some of the amino acids has been lost during evolution. For remembering the names of essential amino acids, there is a mnemonic, PVT TIM HALL, which indicates first letter of name of these amino acids. Thus, essential amino acids as per above sequence are: Phenylalanine, valine, tryptophan, threonine, isoleucine, methionine, histidine, argenine, leucine and lysine.

Essential Amino Acids

It is impossible to maintain equilibrium on diets which are deficient in any one (or more) of these essential amino acids, no matter how much protein is consumed. The term 'essential' is applied to those amino acids needed for tissue replacement and growth, but which cannot be synthesized by the body in amount sufficient to fulfill its normal requirements. They must, therefore, be supplied in the diet, usually combined in protein. A more appropriate term is indispensable amino acids as they differ from other amino acids in being indispensable

Table 9.1: Starting material for synthesis of amino acids				
Glutamate	Oxaloacetate	Pyruvate	Phosphoenol pyruvate	Glycerate 3-phosphate
Glutamate	Aspartate	Alanine	Phenylalanine	Serine
Glutamine	Asparagine	Leucine	Tyrosine	Glycine
Proline	Lysine	Valine	Tryptophan	Cysteine
Arginine	Methionine	Isoleucine		
Histidine	Threonine			

Table 9.2: End products of catabolism of amino acids				
Pyruvate (C₃)	Oxaloacetate (C₄)	α-ketoglutarate (C₅)	Succinyl CoA	Acetyl Coa* and acetoacetyl Coa
Alanine	Aspartate	Glutamate	Methionine	Lysine
Serine	Asparagine	Glutamine	Threonine	Isoleucine
		Proline	Isoleucine	Leucine
Glycine		Arginine	Valine	Tryptophan
Cysteine		Histidine		Phenylalanine
				Tyrosine

* Leucine and lysine are purely ketogenic; other four isoleucine, phenylalanine, tyrosine and tryptophan are both glucogenic as well as ketogenic. Rest 14 amino acids are purely glucogenic.

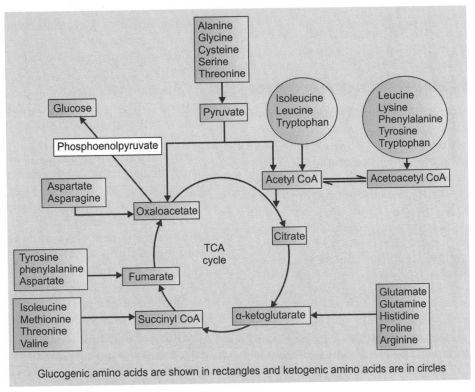

Glucogenic amino acids are shown in rectangles and ketogenic amino acids are in circles

Fig. 9.2: Fates of the carbon skeleton of amino acids

components of the diet. The rest of amino acids can be synthesized in the body by transamination or directly from the essential amino acids.

It has been found that the eight amino acids (phenylalanine, valine, tryptophan, threonine, isoleucine, methionine, leucine and lysine) are indispensable for human adults under normal conditions; exclusion of any one of these essential amino acids leads to negative nitrogen balance. The deficiency signs includes: fatigue, loss of appetite and nervous irritability. When the missing amino acids are added to the diet, perfect health is promptly restored. In addition, histidine and arginine may be required under conditions of growth. The capacity of body to synthesize these two, although adequate for protein maintenance, may not suffice for the more extensive calls of protein accumulation.

Non-essential Amino Acids

The amino acids required for tissue protein synthesis, but which can be synthesized in our body in amount sufficient to fulfill the normal requirement so that body does not depend on dietary supply for them. These are—glycine, alanine, proline, cysteine, aspartic acid, glutamic acid, serine, asparagine, glutamine and tyrosine.

NON-PROTEIN FUNCTION OF AMINO ACIDS

The amino acids have many functions other than making proteins. These are:

1. **Maintenance of immunity:** Amino acids are involved in giving immunity by maintaining the vulnerable surfaces of the body in such a way so as to resist infections. Most of the external agents that cause damage to the human system enter through the (a) lung or (b) gastrointestinal tract. Both these organs are protected by mucus membrane, which offer resistance against the invasion of micro-organism and have the ability to stop the growth of micro-organism. The amino acid which is important and found in mucus membrane is threonine.

2. **Synthesis of glutathione (GSH):** Glutathione (γ-glutamyl cysteinyl glycine) is a tripeptide consisting of three amino acids: (1) Glutamine (2) Cysteine and (3) Glycine. It is necessary to scavenge and quench the free radicals. Many of the age related diseases like loss of memory function, cardio vascular diseases, cancer, etc. can be due to oxidative damage. Glutathione acts as antioxidant.

3. **Glutamine:** It is amide of glutamic acid and is formed to trap ammonia by the kidneys. It is used to neutralize acids by forming ammonium ion.

4. **Taurine:** Taurine is formed from cysteine and it forms bile salt, sodium or potassium taurocholates. The level of taurine in breast milk is higher, providing protective functions from free radicals.

5. **Creatine:** Creatine is formed from three amino acids—glycine, arginine and methionine. The function of creatine as phosphate is to provide quick energy to muscles.

6. **Tyrosine:** Tyrosine amino acid is involved in the biosynthesis of variety of compounds namely, thyroid hormones, dopamine, epinephrine, norepinephrine and melanin.

7. **Tryptophan:** Tryptophan amino acid is utilized for the synthesis of serotonin (neurotransmitter), melatonin and B-complex vitamin, niacin.

8. **Purine ring:** The formation of ring structure of purine, nitrogen bases of nucleic acids, adenine and guanine utilizes the involvement of amino acids glycine, aspartate and glutamine. All the four nitrogen groups in purine ring are from these amino acids.

9. **Arginine:** Nitric oxide (NO) is synthesized from arginine. It is utilized in the treatment of angina pectoris and erectile dysfunction.

10. **Histidine:** Histidine forms histamine which stimulates gastric acid secretion and anti-histaminic drugs are used to control allergic and anaphylactic reactions.

INBORN ERRORS OF AMINO ACIDS

Several inherited inborn disorders are associated with metabolism of amino acids due to enzyme defects. Some of the disorders are listed in Table 9.3.

Table 9.3: Some inborn errors of amino acid metabolism

Inborn errors	Affected amino acids	Defective enzymes
Phenylketonuria	Phenylalanine	Phenylalanine hydroxylase
Alkaptonuria	Tyrosine	Homogentisate oxidase
Albinism	Tyrosine	Tyrosinase
Maple syrup urine disease	Branched chain amino acids	Branched chain α-ketoacids dehydrogenase
Histidinemia	Histidine	Histidase
Hartnup's disease	Tryptophan	Defect in absorption of tryptophan
Cystinuria	Cysteine, lysine, arginine and ornithine	Defect in carrier system for reabsorption of amino acids

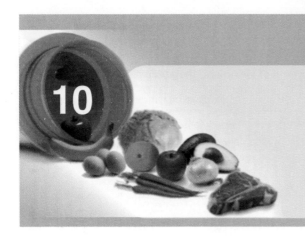

Lipid Metabolism

INTRODUCTION

As you have learnt that the lipids are oil like greasy substances insoluble in water. Our diet and body is abundant in simple lipid— fat, while compound lipids—phospholipids and glycolipids are present in small amount. The derived lipids like cholesterol is found in trace amount. Therefore, we shall discuss metabolism of fats in detail and of rest in brief. An overview of fat metabolism is given in Fig. 10.1.

FAT METABOLISM

Dietary fat: A variety of fat is present in human diet which differs in fatty acid composition.

Table 10.1: Typical fatty acid analysis of some dietary fats of animal and plant origin

Source		Saturated			Unsaturated	
	Other	Palmitic	Stearic	Other	Oleic	Linoleic
Animal Fats						
Lard	1.0	29.8	12.7	5.6	47.8	3.1
Chicken	0.3	25.6	7.0	5.9	39.4	21.8
Butter fat	25.6	25.2	9.2	7.2	29.5	3.6
Beef fat	3.4	29.2	21.0	3.5	41.1	1.8
Vegetable Oils						
Corn	0.1	8.1	2.5	2.9	30.1	56.3
Peanuts	5.9	6.3	4.9	—	61.1	21.8
Cotton seed	2.7	23.4	1.1	2.1	22.9	47.8
Soyabean	1.2	9.8	2.4	7.0	28.9	50.7
		Saturated			Oleic	Linoleic
Sunflower		12.00			—	68.0
Sesame		13.75			42.25	43.75
Coconut		90.50			8.00	1.50
Vanaspati ghee (hydrogenated fat)		61.35			28.35	3.05
Ghee (butter oil)		64.50			33.20	2.60
Safflower		7.0			—	78.0

Thus, we see that:

1. Animal fats contain much more saturated fatty acids than vegetable fats and oils.
2. Amongst vegetable fats, only coconut oil is exceptionally rich in saturated fatty acids.
3. Vegetable oils are generally good sources of polyunsaturated fatty acids.
4. Almost all the fatty acids present in natural fats contain even number of carbon atoms.
5. The amount of fatty acids containing less than C16 is negligible. Most fatty acids contain eighteen carbon atoms.
6. Palmitic and stearic acids are predominant fatty acids in saturated and linoleic and oleic acids in unsaturated.
7. Butter is rich in lower fatty acids.

DIGESTION AND ABSORPTION OF DIETARY LIPIDS

As all lipids are insoluble in water, these have to be solubilised before digestive enzymes can act and absorption in blood stream can occur. This occurs in the small intestine mainly by the emulsifying action of bile salts present in bile. Other emulsifying agents are lecithin (a phospholipid present in food), partial hydrolytic products of lecithin (lysolecithin) and mono and diglycerides derived from dietary fats. Certain physical and mechanical processes also aid in their emulsification, viz. mastication of food in the mouth and peristaltic movements of the small intestine.

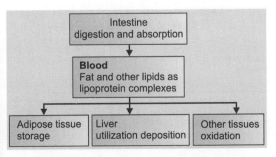

Fig. 10.1: Overview of fat metabolism

Note: Abbreviations used in this chapter

TG: Triglyceride
PL: Phospholipid
FC: Free cholesterol
CE: Cholesterol esters
VLDL: Very low density lipoprotein
LDL: Low density lipoprotein
HDL: High density lipoprotein
CM: Chylomicrons
FA: Fatty acid
P: Proteins
NEFA: Non-esterified fatty acid

The lipids of the food are thus converted into tiny complex molecular aggregates called micelles. All these lipid components are kept soluble by bile salts (Fig. 10.2).

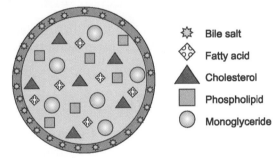

Fig. 10.2: Cross-section of a micelle

Digestion of Fat

Since fat is predominant lipid in the diet, its digestion is discussed here in detail. The fats and oils are digested by hydrolytic enzyme lipase of pancreatic juice. Pancreatic lipase is capable of hydrolyzing ester linkage formed by primary alcoholic group but not of secondary alcoholic group. So the major end product of fat digestion is monoglyceride and free fatty acids. Another enzyme (isomerase) converts –2 glyceride into 1- or 3-monoglyceride which can then be further hydrolyzed into glycerol and fatty acid. This conversion is slow and hence only 25% of total fat is completely hydrolyzed and 75% is incompletely hydrolyzed.

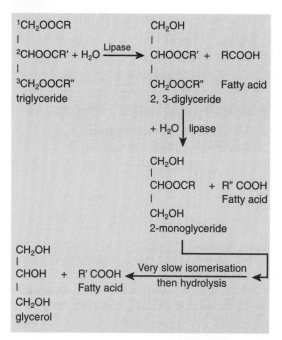

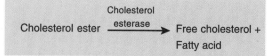

The phospholipids like lecithin are also hydrolyzed to liberate fatty acid from 2-carbon by specific pancreatic enzyme lecithinase.

$$Lecithin \xrightarrow{Lecithinase} Lysolecithin + Fatty\ acid$$

Similarly, the derived lipid–cholesterol, which exists mainly as ester is hydrolyzed to free cholesterol by another pancreatic enzyme, cholesterol esterase.

Absorption

The products of digestion of all the lipids then enter into the mucosal cell. There, they are again reesterified.

i. Mono- or di-glyceride + Fatty acids ⟶ Triglycerides

ii. Lyso lecithin + Fatty acid ⟶ Lecithin

iii. Free cholesterol + Fatty acid ⟶ Cholesterol ester

This reesterification is unique feature of the absorption of lipids. Herein the molecules are first hydrolyzed and then reconstituted before transfer to blood circulation. In contrast, carbohydrates and proteins are absorbed in the form of hydrolyzed product. Secondly, the fatty substances are absorbed by lymphatic system as opposed to water soluble monosaccharides and amino acids, which are passed into portal vein. Therefore, glycerol being water soluble is absorbed by portal venous systems. It is also the route of absorption of water soluble fatty acids of short chains (Fig. 10.3).

The absorbed fatty molecules (TG, PL, CE, C) emerge in the blood plasma as constituent of particles known as chylomicrons

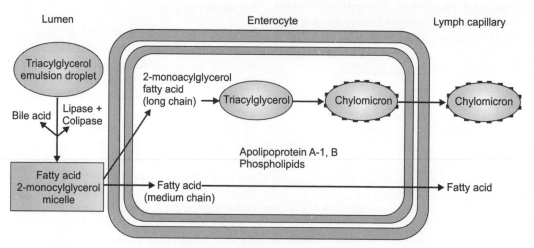

Fig. 10.3: Digestion and absorption of fat

(Fig. 10.4). These are of size, 0.5–1.5 μ. The hydrophobic lipids are rendered hydrophilic by special proteins called apoproteins. These proteins are synthesized in the intestine and are incorporated to form chylomicrons.

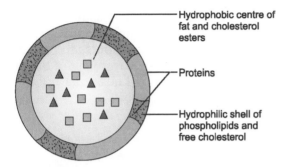

Fig. 10.4: Cross-section of chylomicron

The absorption of lipids begins after one hour of meal, peaks at 2–4 hrs and is completed in 6–10 hrs. Hence, the plasma obtained during post meals is turbid or milky due to presence of chylomicrons. This milkness is gradually cleared by an enzyme present in plasma—lipoprotein lipase. This enzyme breaks triglycerides into glycerol and three fatty acids.

However, there is the difference in digestion and absorption of dietary triacylglycerols and short chain triacylglycerols as illustrated in Fig. 10.5

TRANSPORT OF LIPIDS

All lipid fractions are present in blood all the time but the concentration varies; it is highest during absorptive phase and lowest during post absorptive phase. Table 10.2 gives an idea of average value of fatty constituents in plasma after overnight fast.

The lipids in blood circulation are present as complex with proteins, called lipoproteins. The plasma lipids are contributed

Table 10.2: Post absorptive plasma lipid concentrations (the range of normal variation is very wide)

Lipid fraction	Average concentration (mg/100 ml)
Total	570
Triglycerides	140
Phospholipids	215
Cholesterol	200
NEFA	15

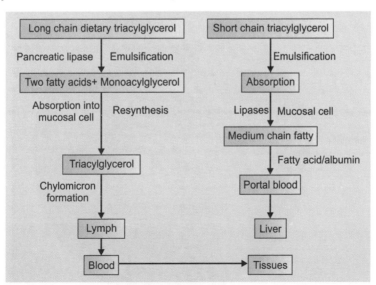

Fig. 10.5: Difference in digestion and absorption of long chain triacylglycerols and short chain triacylglycerols

mainly by intestine by absorption of dietary lipids and are present as chylomicrons and lipoproteins.

The blood lipids are lipids in transit from organ of absorption (intestine) to organ of storage (adipose tissue), organ of utilization (other tissues) and organ of oxidation and deposition in liver and excretion of cholesterol in bile.

Plasma Lipoproteins

The plasma lipoproteins are molecular complexes of lipids and specific proteins called apolipoproteins. They are composed of a neutral lipid core (containing triacylglycerol and cholesteryl ester) surrounded by a shell of apolipoproteins (apoproteins), phospholipids and non-esterified cholesterol all oriented in such a way that their polar portions are exposed on the surface of lipoprotein. This makes the particle soluble in aqueous medium (Fig. 10.6).

Like other cellular constituent, lipoproteins are in a constant state of synthesis, degradation and removal from the plasma.

They keep the lipids soluble in plasma during their transport in them, and to provide an efficient mechanism for delivering their lipid contents to the tissues. In humans, the delivery system is less perfect than in other animals and as a result, human experience a gradual deposition of lipids–especially cholesterol in tissues. This is potentially life threatening occurrence when the lipid deposition contributes to plaque formation, causing the narrowing of blood vessels—a condition known as *atherosclerosis* as shown in Fig. 10.7.

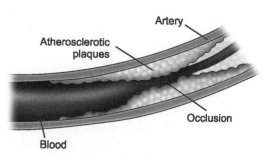

Fig. 10.7: Atherosclerosis

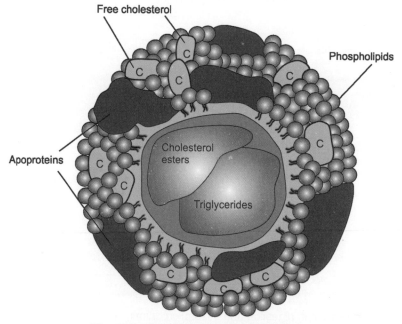

Fig. 10.6: Structure of plasma lipoprotein

SEPARATION OF PLASMA LIPOPROTEINS

The lipoproteins of plasma can be separated into different fractions; mainly two techniques have been used for this purpose—electrophoresis and ultracentrifugation.

Electrophoretic Separation

The presence of proteins in lipoprotein molecule confers electrical charge on it which makes it possible to separate lipoprotein fractions as we do separate plasma or serum proteins. Usually two fractions are separated which are named α and β-lipoproteins as their migration on electrophoregram corresponds to the position of α- and β-globulins of plasma or serum proteins. Sometimes a third band between α- and β-lipoproteins is seen which is termed as pre-β-fraction. This separation has limited utility/applicability (Fig. 10.8).

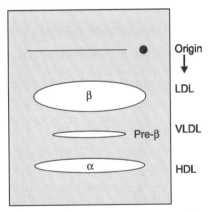

Fig. 10.8: Electrophoretic separation of plasma lipoproteins

Ultracentrifugal Separation

The plasma lipoproteins have been extensively studied using this method of separation. The plasma sample is placed in a tube containing NaCl solution of 1.063 density and is centrifuged at a very high speed in a centrifuge called ultracentrifuge. The various particles of lipoproteins separate based upon their density. The lower the density of lipoprotein particles, the faster the upward migration. On the other hand, the higher the density, the faster is the downward movement of the particles. It may be noted that the density of the particle is determined by the relative proportion of protein and lipids. The lipids are lighter than water and the proteins are heavier, so the greater the amount of proteins, the higher will be the density. Conversely, the greater the quantity of lipids (especially TG), the lower will be the density (Fig. 10.9).

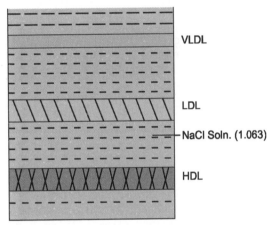

Fig. 10.9: Ultracentrifugal separation of plasma lipoproteins

Normally, the following fractions are obtained on ultracentrifugation of plasma–very low density lipoproteins (VLDL), low density lipoproteins (LDL) and high density lipoproteins (HDL). LDL and HDL roughly represents to α- and β-lipoprotein fractions obtained on electrophoresis. The plasma collected during absorptive phase also contains chylomicron (density 0.96) at the top of the tube. The details of these fractions of lipoproteins are given in Table 10. 3.

1. **Chylomicrons** (density 0.96): The chylomicrons separate out from plasma obtained after a fatty meal. This represents fat derived from intestinal

Table 10. 3: Approximate chemical composition of plasma lipoproteins

	Proteins	Phospholipids	Free cholesterol	Cholesterol esters	Trigly-cerides
Chylomicrons	1	10	—	0–10	80–90
VLDL	10	15	—	15	60
LDL	20	20	10	40	0–10
HDL	45	30	5	20	0

absorption in transit to storage depots. It contains 1% protein, 99% lipid, (triglycerides, phospholipids and cholesterol).

Function: Its function is to carry dietary acylglycerols.

2. **Very low density lipoproteins (VLDL)** (density 0.96–1.006): The fatty components from liver are transported as VLDL and LDL. VLDL is rich in triglycerides while LDL in cholesterol. It represents pre β-lipoprotein on electrophoresis.

Function: VLDL's function is to carry endogenously made triacylglycerol and cholesterol.

3. **Low density lipoproteins (LDL)** (density 1.006–1.063): These are synthesized by liver and contain about 3/4 of serum cholesterol. It corresponds to β-lipoprotein on electrophoretic separation.

Function: Its function is to carry cholesterol and cholesterol esters.

4. **High density lipoproteins (HDL)** (density 1.063–1.21): These contain low percentage of triglycerides and cholesterol, same amount of phospholipid, but more protein. It is actually α-lipoprotein function obtained on electrophoresis of plasma/serum.

Function: It functions in reverse cholesterol transport and exchange of apolipoprotein.

5. **Very high density lipoproteins (VHDL) or Albumin - FFA complex** (99% albumin and 1% FFA): This represents greatest amount of lipid transported in blood. Almost 25–30 molecules of free fatty acids are present in combination with a molecule of albumin. These free fatty acids are mainly derived from adipose tissue; are metabolically most active and have a half life of 2–3 minutes, so this fraction cannot be demonstrated by electrophoresis or ultracentrifugation.

CATABOLISM OF FAT

The dietary fat as well as fat stored in adipose tissues can be catabolized completely to give energy. As already mentioned, fat is most concentrated source of energy; 2¼ times that of carbohydrates or proteins.

The fat has to be first hydrolyzed to liberate constituent glycerol and fatty acids before further catabolism can proceed. This is accomplished by the enzyme lipase—lipoprotein lipase in plasma for splitting TG of lipoprotein particles and adipose tissue lipase in adipose tissue for stored TG (Fig. 10.10). This enzyme is under the control of hormones—epinephrine, norepinephrine and glucagon.

These two lipases differ from pancreatic lipase in their ability to hydrolyze all the three ester bonds (primary as well as secondary).

Triglyceride $\xrightarrow{\text{Lipase}}$ Glycerol + 3 fatty acids

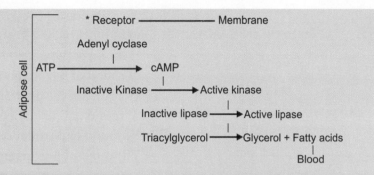

Hormone *(adrenalin, glucagon, ACTH) binds to membrane receptor and activates membrane bound enzyme adenyl cyclase which produces cAMP from ATP. cAMP converts inactive kinase into active kinase; the latter catalyse the conversion of inactive lipase into active lipase by phosphorylation. The active lipase finally completely hydrolyzes triacylglycerol into glycerol and three fatty acids, which leave the adipose cell to enter blood .

Fig. 10.10: Lipolysis

CATABOLISM OF GLYCEROL

Glycerol liberated by mobilization of fat in adipose tissue cannot be used for resynthesis of triglycerides as enzyme glycerokinase is absent there. Since glycerol is water soluble, it is rapidly transferred to liver or other tissues for further utilization. It can be activated by glycerokinase to form glycerol-3-phosphate to combine with fatty acids to form neutral fat.

CH$_2$OH $\quad$ ATP $\quad$ ADP $\quad$ CH$_2$OH
CHOH $\xrightarrow{\text{Glycerol kinase}}$ CHOH
CH$_2$OH $\qquad\qquad\qquad$ CH$_2$O~P

Glycerol $\qquad\qquad$ Glycerol-3-phosphate

NAD $\quad$ NADH$_2$ $\quad$ CH$_2$OH
$\xrightarrow{\hspace{2cm}}$ C=O
Glycerol-3-phosphate $\quad$ CH$_2$O~(P)
dehydrogenase

Dihydroxy acetone phosphate

Alternatively, it can form dihydroxyl acetone phosphate and thus enter into glycolytic pathway (of carbohydrates) for energy production. Thus, it may be noted that glycerol, although a constituent of fats and other lipids, it much more resembles carbohydrates, chemically as well as metabolically. Its structure resembles monosaccharides (e.g. glucose), it is also water soluble like them and is catabolized like them in glycolysis.

CATABOLISM OF FATTY ACIDS

Fatty acids liberated by hydrolysis of depot fat in the adipose tissue are transferred to other tissues after binding with albumin of plasma. Free fatty acid—albumin complex is metabolically most active. One albumin molecule can bind as many as 25–30 molecules of fatty acids. Their half life in plasma is only 2–3 minutes.

Fatty acids are completely oxidized into liver and other tissues. The most important and well known pathway of fatty acid oxidation is β-oxidation pathway. Dietary fat is mainly composed of saturated fatty acids of even carbon number. In this category, palmitic (C$_{16}$) and stearic (C$_{18}$) acids are predominant fatty acids. Hence β-oxidation pathway will be described here taking palmitic acid as an example. The enzymes of this pathway occur in the mitochondria. It is active in many tissues liver, heart, kidney, muscle, lung, brain and adipose tissue.

β-oxidation Pathway

β-oxidation pathway is the sequential removal of two carbon units (C$_2$ units) as

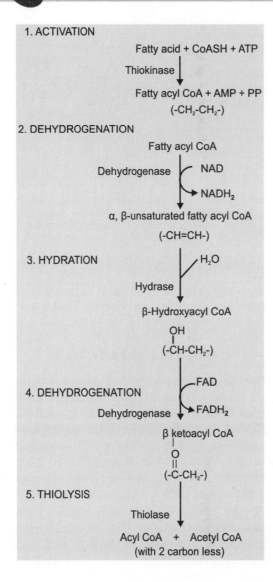

1. ACTIVATION

Fatty acid + CoASH + ATP

Thiokinase

Fatty acyl CoA + AMP + PP

($-CH_2-CH_2-$)

2. DEHYDROGENATION

Fatty acyl CoA

Dehydrogenase — NAD

→ $NADH_2$

α, β-unsaturated fatty acyl CoA

($-CH=CH-$)

3. HYDRATION

H_2O

Hydrase

β-Hydroxyacyl CoA

OH
|
($-CH-CH_2-$)

4. DEHYDROGENATION

FAD

Dehydrogenase → $FADH_2$

β ketoacyl CoA
|
O
||
($-C-CH_2-$)

5. THIOLYSIS

Thiolase

Acyl CoA + Acetyl CoA
(with 2 carbon less)

Palmitic acid (C_{16}), after

I round of β-oxidation – Fatty acid $C_{14} + C_2$

II round of β-oxidation-$C_{12} + C_2$

III round of β-oxidation-$C_{10} + C_2$

IV round of β-oxidation-$C_8 + C_2$

V round of β-oxidation-$C_6 + C_2$

VI round of β-oxidation-$C_4 + C_2$

VII round of β-oxidation-$C_2 + C_2$

Energetics

One turn of β-oxidation liberates one $NADH_2$ and one $FADH_2$. The hydrogen transfer from these on ETC will produce 3 and 2 ATP, respectively (Total 5 ATP). Since palmitic acid will undergo β-oxidation seven times, so $7 \times 5 = 35$ ATP will be produced on this account. Further palmitic acid produces eight molecules of acetyl CoA by breakdown in β-oxidation which would on complete oxidation in TCA cycle produce $12 \times 8 = 96$ molecules of ATP. Thus, total no. of ATP produced from palmitic acid is $35 + 96 = 131$ ATP. Since both the high energy bonds of ATP were consumed in initial activation of fatty acid, the net energy production from palmitic acid is $131 - 2 = 129$ ATP molecules.

ANABOLISM

The synthesis of fat requires three fatty acid molecules and glycerol. The fatty acids are completely synthesized from basic unit— acetyl CoA (C_2). The sequential addition of these C_2 units gives the fatty acid of desired chain length. One of the important sources of C_2 units is pyruvate (oxidative decarboxylation of pyruvate) which is the end product of glucose breakdown. The glycerol moiety is furnished by glycolysis, i.e. dihydroxy acetone phosphate. This will combine with fatty acid to give fat. Thus, carbohydrates are easily converted into fat and deposited in the body. Therefore, it is said that excess of carbohydrates is fattening.

acetyl coenzyme A. This pathway has five steps. The initial step is the activation of fatty acid molecule.

Acetyl CoA is diverted to TCA cycle for complete oxidation. The original fatty acid is now shortened by two carbons and is in activated state (acyl CoA), hence, the process is repeated from steps 2 to 5. The repetition of this pathway seven times will produce eight molecules of acetyl CoA from the palmitic acid.

SYNTHESIS OF FATTY ACIDS

One of the method by which fatty acids are synthesized is by reversal of β-oxidation pathway as most of the enzymes are reversible. This occurs in the mitochondria. Another pathway also exists outside the mitochondria, which is more important.

Extra Mitochondrial Pathway

This system has been found in many tissues including liver, kidney, lungs, mammary glands and adipose tissue. It converts acetyl CoA to free palmitate. Its co-factor requirements include NADH, ATP, Mn^{+2} and HCO_3 (as a source of CO_2). Its steps are:

1. Carboxylation

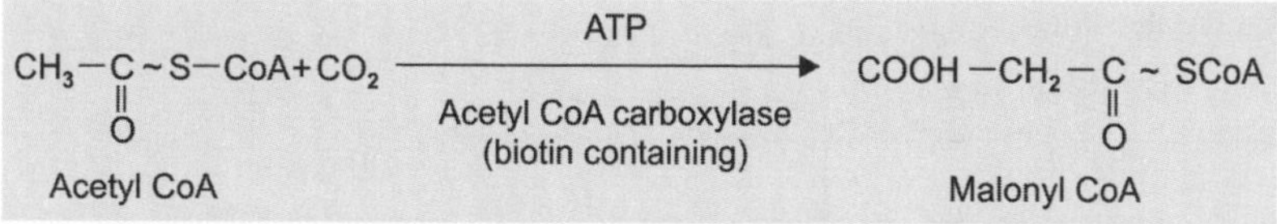

$$CH_3-\underset{\underset{O}{\|}}{C}\sim S-CoA + CO_2 \xrightarrow[\substack{\text{Acetyl CoA carboxylase}\\\text{(biotin containing)}}]{ATP} COOH-CH_2-\underset{\underset{O}{\|}}{C}\sim SCoA$$

Acetyl CoA → Malonyl CoA

2. Transfer to acyl carrier protein (ACP). ACP is combination of enzyme proteins instead of individual enzymes. It has two SH groups, one central group and other peripheral group.

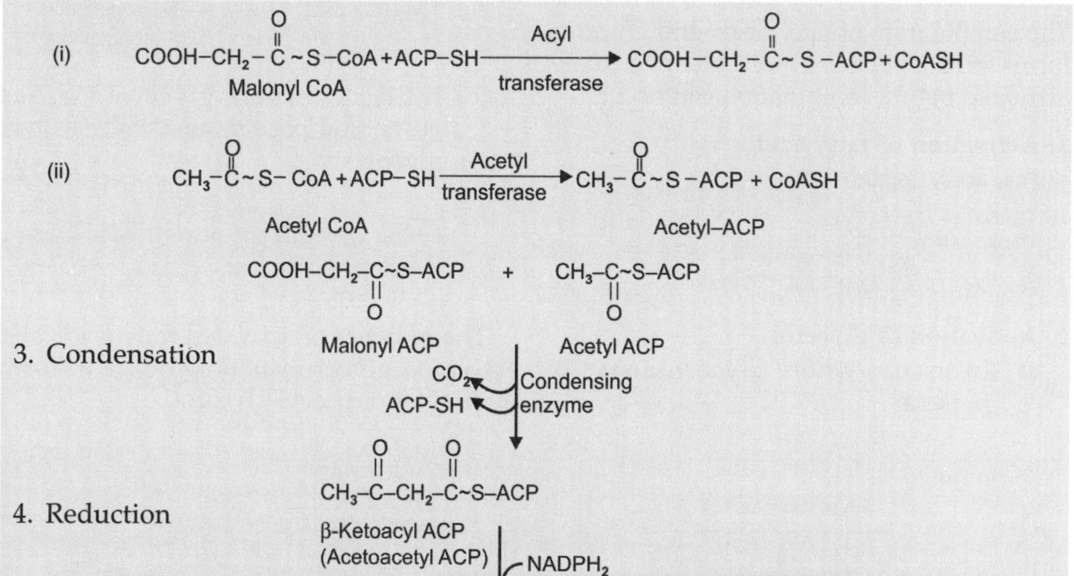

(i) $$COOH-CH_2-\underset{\underset{O}{\|}}{C}\sim S-CoA + ACP-SH \xrightarrow[\text{transferase}]{\text{Acyl}} COOH-CH_2-\underset{\underset{O}{\|}}{C}\sim S-ACP + CoASH$$

Malonyl CoA

(ii) $$CH_3-\underset{\underset{O}{\|}}{C}\sim S-CoA + ACP-SH \xrightarrow[\text{transferase}]{\text{Acetyl}} CH_3-\underset{\underset{O}{\|}}{C}\sim S-ACP + CoASH$$

Acetyl CoA → Acetyl–ACP

$$COOH-CH_2-\underset{\underset{O}{\|}}{C}\sim S-ACP \quad + \quad CH_3-\underset{\underset{O}{\|}}{C}\sim S-ACP$$

3. Condensation

Malonyl ACP   Acetyl ACP

$$\xrightarrow[\substack{CO_2\\ACP\text{-}SH}]{\text{Condensing enzyme}}$$

$$CH_3-\underset{\underset{O}{\|}}{C}-CH_2-\underset{\underset{O}{\|}}{C}-S-ACP$$

4. Reduction

β-Ketoacyl ACP (Acetoacetyl ACP)

$$\xrightarrow[\substack{NADPH_2\\NADP}]{} \quad \text{β-Ketoacyl ACP reductase}$$

$$CH_3-\underset{\underset{OH}{|}}{CH}-CH_2-\underset{\underset{O}{\|}}{C}\sim S-ACP$$

5. Dehydration

β-hyroxyacyl ACP

$$\xrightarrow[\text{Hydrase}]{H_2O}$$

(Contd.)

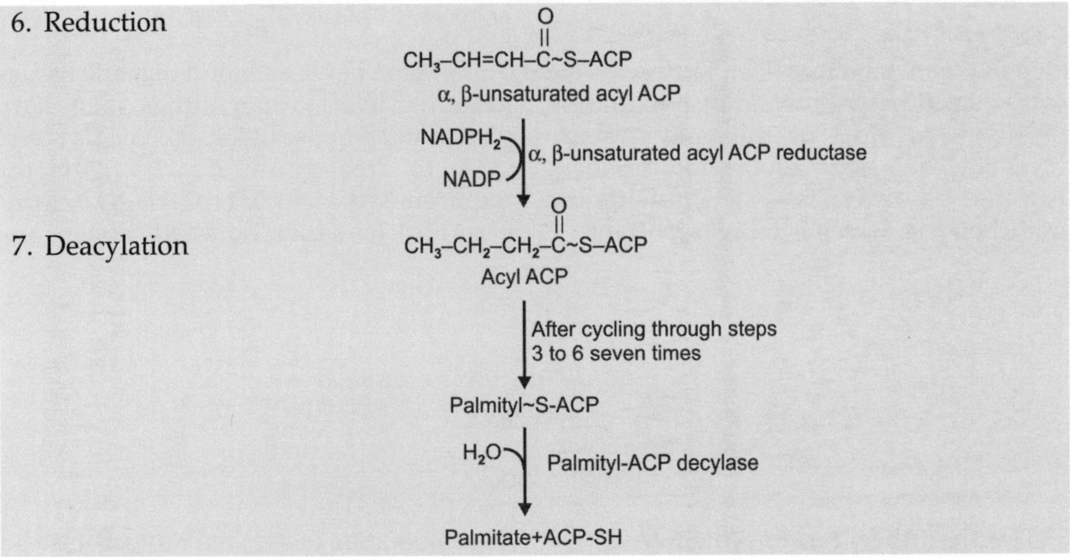

6. Reduction

$$CH_3–CH=CH–\overset{\overset{\displaystyle O}{\|}}{C}–S\sim ACP$$

α, β-unsaturated acyl ACP

NADPH$_2$ ⟍
NADP ⟋ α, β-unsaturated acyl ACP reductase

7. Deacylation

$$CH_3–CH_2–CH_2–\overset{\overset{\displaystyle O}{\|}}{C}\sim S–ACP$$

Acyl ACP

After cycling through steps 3 to 6 seven times

Palmityl~S-ACP

H$_2$O ⟍ Palmityl-ACP decylase

Palmitate+ACP-SH

SYNTHESIS OF FAT (TRIGLYCERIDES)

The combination of fatty acids and glycerol forms fat. Both of these molecules need to be activated before combination can occur.

1. Activation of fatty acid

Fatty acid + CoASH + ATP

Thiokinase ↓

Fatty acyl CoA + AMP + PP

2. Activation of glycerol

(a) In tissues where glycerokinase is present:

$$\text{Glycerol + ATP} \xrightarrow{\text{Glycerokinase}} \alpha\text{-glycero-phosphate}$$

(b) In tissues where glycerokinase is absent (adipose tissues, muscles) via glycolysis:

$$\text{Dihydroxyacetone phosphate} \xrightarrow{\text{Reduction}} \alpha\text{-glycerol phosphate}$$

The moieties of activated fatty acids and activated glycerol then combine to form neutral fat or triacyl glycerol.

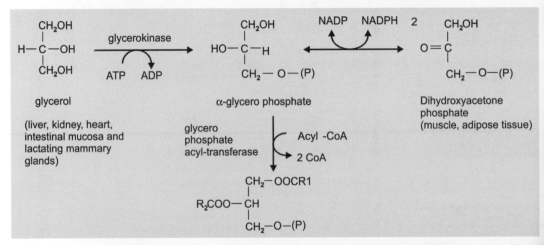

glycerol

(liver, kidney, heart, intestinal mucosa and lactating mammary glands)

α-glycero phosphate

glycero phosphate acyl-transferase

Dihydroxyacetone phosphate
(muscle, adipose tissue)

(Contd..

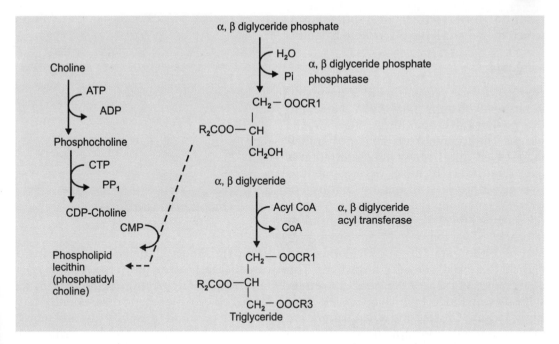

SYNTHESIS OF PHOSPHOLIPIDS

The above pathway also affords for the synthesis of phospholipids. For example, lecithin is synthesized after diglyceride is formed as shown above.

(i) Choline + ATP ⟶ Choline phosphate + ADP

(ii) CTP + Choline Phosphate ⟶ CDP-choline

(iii) Diglyceride + CDP-choline ⟶

FA ⟍
    ⟍ (Glycerol-phosphate-choline)
    ⟋ (Lecithin)
FA ⟋

Pathology

An excess catabolism of fatty acids in β-oxidation pathway, in absence of normal carbohydrate metabolism, usually results into a pathologic state known as Ketosis and occasionally in 'fatty liver'. These occur in starvation and advanced untreated diabetes mellitus.

Ketosis

When acetyl CoA is produced by β-oxidation at a rate much greater than what can be oxidized in TCA cycle, two moles combine to form aceto acetic acid in the liver.

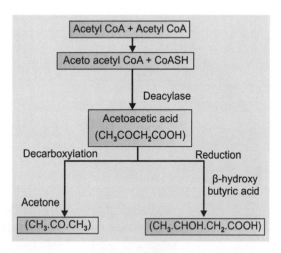

These three compounds are collectively, known as 'Ketone bodies'. Their accumulation in blood is known as 'Ketonemia' and excretion in urine is known as 'Ketonuria'. The condition is described as 'Ketosis'. This condition is dangerous as these are strong acids which cause acidosis (ketoacidosis) and excretion of these acids requires loss of essential ions–sodium and potassium, which may disturb the electrolyte balance.

Fatty Liver

Another disease caused due to abnormality in fat metabolism is 'fatty liver'. Normally liver contains fat in amount less than 5% of its weight. The accumulation of fat greater than this is called 'fatty liver' or fatty infiltration of liver (Fig. 10.11). It causes derangement in liver functions and ultimately cirrhosis of liver which is fatal (Fig. 10.12). 'Fatty liver' occurs when there is much greater influx of fatty acid in liver than what it can incorporate into phospholipids Chronic alcoholics and high fat diet usually develop 'fatty liver'. The other causes of it are of deficiency of certain substances in the diet which are called 'lipotropic factors'. Choline and ethanolamine are most important, lipotropic factors. It is the amino acid methionine which helps in endogenous synthesis of choline by transmethylation reaction (supplying methyl

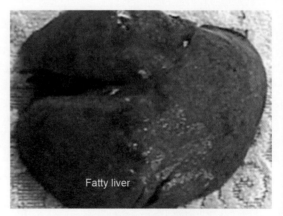

Fig. 10.11: Fatty liver

groups). Dietary deficiency of proteins or essential fatty acids may also predispose to fatty liver by depriving methionine in the former case. In the second case, essential fatty acids are required to esterify glycerol moiety in phospholipid molecule. Prolonged starvation and advanced untreated diabetes mellitus which causes ketosis are also likely to cause fatty liver.

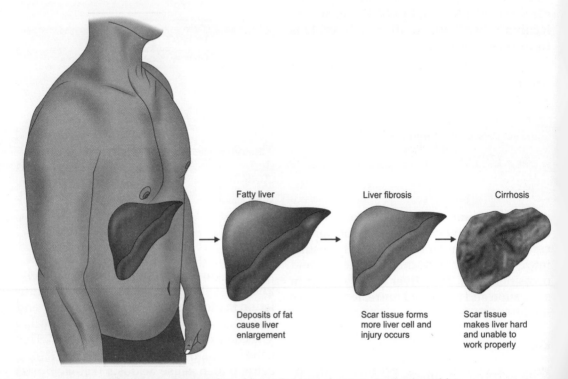

Fig. 10.12: Progression of liver diseases due to necrotization of fat

METABOLISM OF PHOSPHOLIPIDS

There are a number of phospholipids. Lecithin is the chief phospholipid in diet. It may be absorbed as such or after hydrolysis. Phospholipids are digested and absorbed together with fat. Similarly, these are transported as a part of plasma lipoproteins. In tissues, these are synthesized by reaction which is similar to those for fat synthesis except for the some steps. All these aspects have been already described in earlier discussion of fat metabolism.

METABOLISM OF CHOLESTEROL

Introduction

The cholesterol is most important steroid and derived lipid. It has an alcoholic group, hence exists as free and in ester form. It is universal constituent of animal cell. It is also present in plasma membrane to which it imparts fluidity. The metabolism of cholesterol has become important because of its role in causing heart disease and gall stones.

Digestion, Absorption and Transport

The dietary cholesterol comes from animal food; the most important of them is egg. Average daily intake of cholesterol is 0.3 g/day. In the diet, it is mostly present as ester, which is hydrolyzed by pancreatic enzyme, cholesterol esterase, and is reesterified in the mucosal cell. It is present as a part of plasma lipoproteins in free state as well as esterified cholesterol. 70% of plasma cholesterol is transported in β-lipoproteins and 30% in α-lipoproteins. All these aspects have been already described.

Biosynthesis

All tissues are capable of synthesizing cholesterol essentially by the same pathway but the major contributors are liver followed by the intestine. The only raw material needed is acetyl CoA. The cholesterol biosynthetic pathway is very lengthy and complicated, so we shall present only outline. The complete cholesterol ($C_{27}H_{46}O$) molecule is made from a number of molecules of acetyl CoA (C_2). All other steroid compounds are then synthesized from cholesterol.

Main Steps of Cholesterol Biosynthesis

1. Synthesis of mevalonate from acetate (6 C compounds by condensing three units of 2 C compounds).
2. Synthesis of isoprenoid by decarboxylation of mevalonate (5 C from 6 C by removing one C as CO_2).
3. Synthesis of farnesyl pyro phosphate (15 C) from three 5 C compounds.
4. Synthesis of squalene (30 C) by condensing two molecules of 15 C.
5. Final steps include: Cyclisation of squalene followed by three demethylations (30 C–3 C = 27 C).

Slight variations in the sequence of final steps give different pathway for synthesis.

Principal precursors of cholesterol are desmosterol and 7-dehydrocholesterol.

Plasma Cholesterol

The plasma cholesterol is quite variable. It depends upon body weight, sex, race and show diurnal and seasonal variations. Its normal value is taken as 150–250 mg/100 ml. In plasma, it exists in two forms—free and esterified. 60–80% is esterified and 20–40% is free cholesterol. Plasma cholesterol is mainly endogenously synthesized and contribution of dietary cholesterol is much less. Liver synthesizes cholesterol as well as esterifies it, so in liver diseases, a decrease in plasma cholesterol with selective reduction in esterified fraction is noticed.

Cholesterol is excreted through intestine as such and after conversion into bile acids and bile salts in the liver.

Hypocholesterolemia

The most important hormone affecting plasma cholesterol is thyroid hormone. It has inverse relationship, so hypercholesterolemia is observed in hypothyroidism and hypocholesterolemia in hyperthyroidism. Hypocholesterolemia is also seen in malnutrition, anemia and chronic infections.

Hypercholesterolemia

Apart from hypothyroidism, hypercholesterolemia is sometimes seen in diabetes mellitus and essentially in nephrotic syndrome and obstructive jaundice. In the former case, it is due to loss in urine of enzyme lipoprotein lipase, together with proteins which clears plasma of TG, CE and other lipids. In obstructive jaundice, the increase is due to inability to excrete it in intestine.

Cholesterol Metabolism in Liver

Liver is the main organ of synthesis metabolism and synthesis of cholesterol as shown in Fig. 10.13.

Diseases

The elevated plasma cholesterol usually causes atherosclerosis while the cholesterol in bile sometimes precipitates as gall stones.

These two are important diseases related to cholesterol metabolism and their incidence is increasing in modern times. It is always desirable to reduce elevated cholesterol by drugs as it alters the course of atherosclerotic process or precipitation in gall bladder. Some such drugs are D-thyroxine, nicotinic acid, probunol, cholestyramine, clofibrate and colestipol.

ATHEROSCLEROSIS

Atherosclerosis is a condition in which there is deposition of lipids, blood and blood products and calcium salts in the arteries (Fig. 10.7) associated with medical changes. Cholesterol and other lipids are insoluble in aqueous medium. However, they are solubilized in the blood by forming hydrophilic complexes with protein, called lipoprotein. Nevertheless, some deposition of fatty material does take place in the lumen of arteries right from the birth and this goes on with advancing age. This, in due course of time, may become as large as to physically obstruct the blood supply to the concerned organ (Fig. 10.14).

There are several other factors which may hasten or aid this deposition, causing partial or complete blockade of the arteries. These are platelet aggregation and thrombin formation. If any of the coronary arteries is

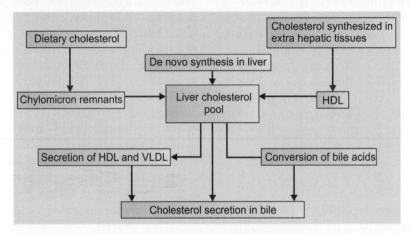

Fig.10.13: Cholesterol metabolism in liver

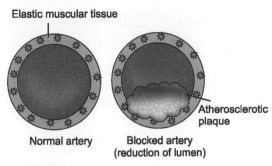

Elastic muscular tissue

Normal artery

Blocked artery
(reduction of lumen)

Atherosclerotic plaque

Fig. 10.14: Cross-section of normal and blocked artery

blocked, it would cause damage to the affected myocardium. This is called heart attack or myocardial infarction and is one of the major killers in the world. If blood supply to the brain is affected, it causes stroke. Both the conditions have serious consequences.

GALL STONES

Cholesterol is an important constituent of bile along with bile salts. It is insoluble in water, but has a very low solubility in presence of bile salts. Whenever it is present in higher concentration than that which can

be solubilized, the precipitation occurs in the form of microcrystals. The continued growth of these crystals gives rise to stone like substances, called gall stones (Fig. 10.15). Hence, cholesterol is the universal constituent of human gall stones.

Gall stone formation is believed to be initiated by first formation of a nucleus of calcium bilirubinate which is derived from the hydrolysis of bilirubin diglucuronides (also present in bile). The presence of stones in gall bladder may cause pain, obstruct the free flow of bile, damage the gall bladder wall and hence, may have to be removed surgically.

HYPERLIPOPROTEINEMIA

The term hyperlipoproteinemia describes a group of disorders in which serum lipoprotein levels are abnormally elevated. Diet also affects the development of hyperlipoproteinemias. The dietary factors causing an increase in plasma lipoprotein in a great many people are obesity and high intake of food rich in cholesterol and saturated fats. Table 10.4 depicts different types of hyperlipoproteinemias.

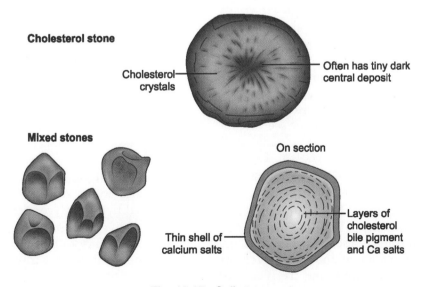

Cholesterol stone

Cholesterol crystals

Often has tiny dark central deposit

Mixed stones

On section

Thin shell of calcium salts

Layers of cholesterol bile pigment and Ca salts

Fig. 10.15: Gall stones

Table 10.4: Types of hyperlipoproteinemia

Type	Triglycerides	Total cholesterol	LDL cholesterol	Raised lipoproteins
I	+++	+	N	Chylomicrons
IIa	N	++	++	LDL
IIb	++	++	++	LDL/VLDL
III	++	+	N	Chylomicrons
IV	++	N/+	N	VLDL
V	++	+	N	VLDL/chylomicrons

N: normal; +: slightly raised; ++: moderately raised; +++: extremely raised

Types of Hyperlipoproteinemia

a. *Type I* is an uncommon pattern marked by elevated chylomicrons. Cholesterol is normal and triglyceride is markedly elevated, usually greater than 1000 mg/dl.

b. *Type IIa* is marked by high LDL with normal VLDL. The genetic disorder associated with this pattern is familial hypercholesterolemia, in which there is an autosomal dominant pattern of inheritance. The biochemical defect is a deficiency of LDL receptors. This pattern is also seen secondary to nephritic syndrome, Cushing's syndrome and hypothyroidism.

c. *Type IIb* is a common pattern characterized by increases of LDL and VLDL. Both cholesterol and triglycerides are elevated. Familial combined hyperlipoproteinemia, also called familial multiple lipoproteins – type hyperlipidemia, is an order in which individual with type II a, type II b and type IV hyperlipoproteinemia are found in the same family. Type II b can be seen secondary to nephrotic syndrome, Cushing's diseases and hypothyroidism. Primary type II b can be aggravated by exogenous obesity or glucocorticoid.

d. *Type III* is marked by reduced electrophoretic mobility of VLDL. In this, cholesterol and triglycerides are both elevated, frequently to about the same level, for example, cholesterol and triglycerides both may be 400 mg/dl. The primary form of this disorder is called familial dysbetalipoproteinemia. These patients accumulate partially degraded VLDL.

e. *Type IV* is a common pattern of hyperlipoproteinemia. It is marked by elevated VLDL with high cholesterol and triglycerides.

• The primary disorders associated with this pattern are familial multiple lipoprotein–type hyperlipidemia and the mild form of familial hypertriglyceridemia.

• In other associated disorder, elevated VLDL is common secondary to diabetes and uremia, and also associated with hyperpituitarism and nephritic syndrome. Alcohol, glucocorticoid, oestrogen and exogenous obesity may aggravate an already elevated VLDL in patient with primary hyperlipidemia but they seldom induce hyperlipidemia in normal individual.

f. *Type V*, a rare pattern, is marked by elevated chylomicrons and VLDL. Both triglycerides and cholesterols are high.

• The primary disorders with the pattern are familial lipoprotein lipase deficiency, apolipoprotein C II deficiency and the more severe form of the familial hypertriglyceridemias.

• Type V hyperlipoproteinemia may be seen secondary to the same disorders as type IV, it is most commonly seen secondary to poorly controlled diabetes.

Chemistry and Metabolism of Nucleic Acids

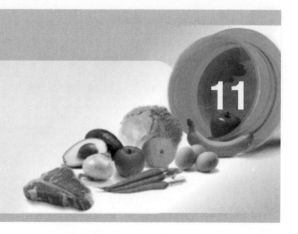

11

INTRODUCTION

Nucleoproteins are one of the groups of conjugated proteins. They contain a nucleic acid molecule attached to one or more molecules of a simple protein. They have very important role in heredity, genetics, protein synthesis, mutation, viral infections, cancer and genetic engineering.

Like carbohydrates and proteins, the complex molecules of nucleic acids are made up of simple molecules. In order to understand nucleoprotein architecture, the molecule is hydrolyzed and the hydrolytic products are studied.

HYDROLYSIS OF NUCLEOPROTEIN

The stepwise hydrolysis of a nucleoprotein by acid yields the following simple substances.

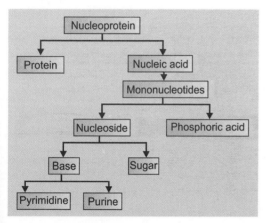

Thus, a molecule of nucleoprotein contains a nucleic acid and simple protein.

The simple protein is usually a basic protein, such as a protamine or histone, because nucleic acid molecules are acidic.

Let us see the structure of these compounds.

Phosphoric Acid

Phosphoric acid present in nucleic acid is ortho-phosphoric acid (H_3PO_4). Its structure is:

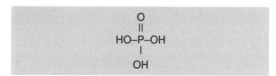

All the three OH groups are acidic and can react to alcoholic groups to form ester linkage.

Sugars

A pentose sugar is present in a nucleic acid molecule. It may be either a ribose or deoxyribose. The resulting nucleic acid is, therefore, called a ribonucleic acid (RNA) or deoxyribonucleic acid (DNA), respectively. Deoxyribose ($C_5H_{10}O_4$) differs from ribose ($C_5H_{10}O_5$) in having one oxygen atom less at carbon number 2.

All the hydroxyl groups in these two sugars are capable of reacting with suitable compounds such as acids.

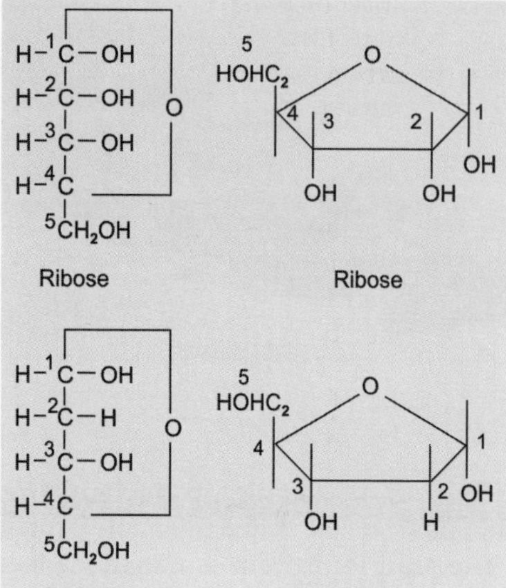

Ribose

Ribose

Deoxyribose

Deoxyribose

with numbering according to the International System. Nucleic acids contain two pyrimidines—cytosine and either uracil or thymine (methyl uracil). RNA contains uracil but DNA contains thymine.

Purines: The purine bases have two heterocyclic rings—one as that of pyrimidine, which is fused to a five membered nitrogenous ring. The numbering of atoms is shown below. The two purines which occur commonly in the nucleic acids are adenine and guanine. Other purines of interest are uric acid, xanthine and hypoxanthine.

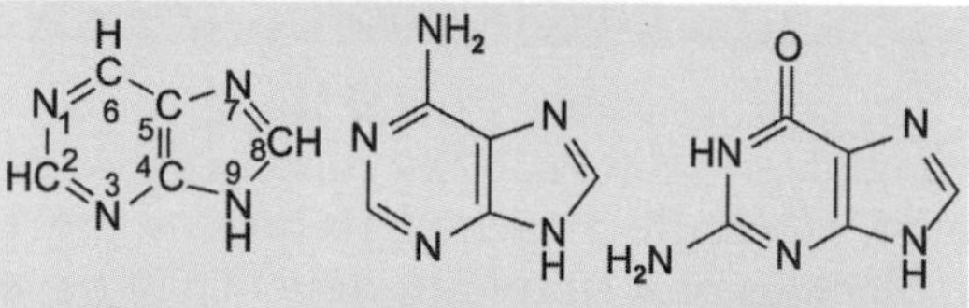

Purine

Adenine

Guanine

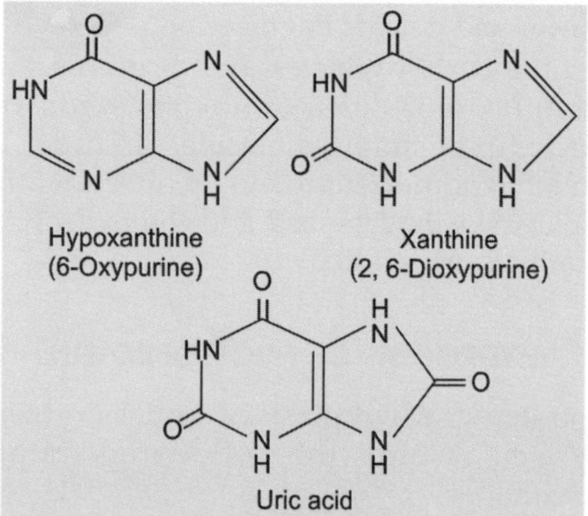

Bases

The nitrogenous bases of nucleic acids belong to either a pyrimidine or a purine group.

Pyrimidines: Pyrimidine is a six-membered heterocyclic ring. It is shown here

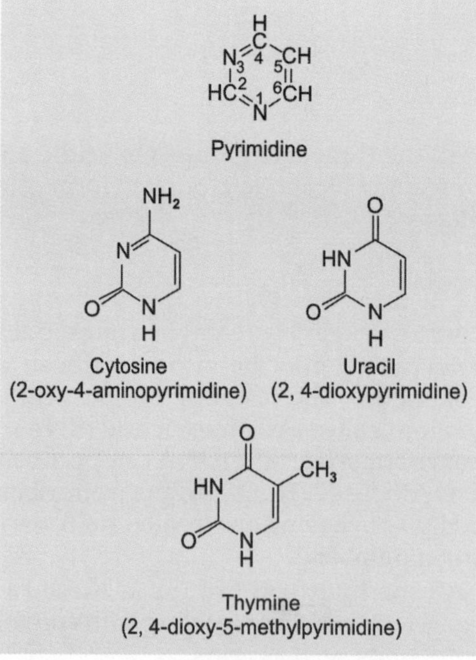

Hypoxanthine
(6-Oxypurine)

Xanthine
(2, 6-Dioxypurine)

Uric acid
(2, 6, 8-Trioxypurine)

Pyrimidine

Cytosine
(2-oxy-4-aminopyrimidine)

Uracil
(2, 4-dioxypyrimidine)

Thymine
(2, 4-dioxy-5-methylpyrimidine)

Tautomerism is shown by uric acid and other oxypurines and oxypyrimidines. Purine and pyrimidine also form salts because nitrogen is weakly basic:

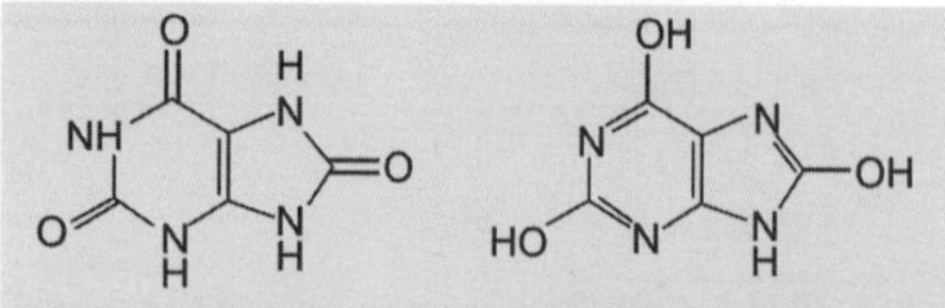

Uric acid (ketoform)

Uric acid (enol form) forms salt with alkali

Nucleosides

Nucleosides are formed by linking of purine or pyrimidine base to the sugar. Bases are linked to sugar at 1 position of pyrimidine and 9 position of purine. The hydrogen at these positions forms water with hydroxylic group at carbon number 1 of pentose sugar. Some common nucleosides are:

Nucleosides		Bases		Sugars
Adenosine	=	Adenine	+	Ribose
Guanosine	=	Guanine	+	Ribose
Cytidine	=	Cytosine	+	Ribose
Uridine	=	Uracil	+	Ribose
Thymidine	=	Thymine	+	Deoxy ribose

Nucleotides

When a nucleoside reacts with ortho-phosphoric acid, a nucleotide is formed. The phosphate is attached to sugar at carbon 5 by an ester bond with elimination of a molecule of water. The names and composition of some common nucleotides are given below:

Nucleotides		Bases		Sugars		Acids
Adenylic acid	=	Adenine	+	Ribose	+	Phosphoric acid
Guanylic acid	=	Guanine	+	Ribose	+	Phosphoric acid
Cytidylic acid	=	Cytosine	+	Ribose	+	Phosphoric acid
Uridylic acid	=	Uracil	+	Ribose	+	Phosphoric acid
Thymidilic acid	=	Thymine	+	Deoxyribose	+	Phosphoric acid

Uridylic acid

Adenosine-5'-monophosphate (AMP)
Adenosine-5'-diphosphate (ADP)
Adenosine-5'-triphosphate (ATP)

POLYNUCLEOTIDES OR NUCLEIC ACIDS

A large number of nucleotides combine to form what is known as polynucleotide-(Base-sugar-phosphoric acid)$_n$, just as a large number of monosaccharide glucose, combine to form a polysaccharide with establishment of a glycosidic bond between two neighbouring sugar units. The high molecular weight nucleic acids are polynucleotides in which the phosphate residues of each nucleotide act as bridges in forming diesters. Their structure is represented below in the simplest form, where B represents base, S stands for sugar and P denotes phosphoric acid.

(3' end)

B—S—P

B—S—P

B—S—P

B—S

(5' end)

The carbon atoms of pentose are numbered 1′, 2′, 3′, 4′ and 5′ to distinguish from atom numbers of the base. Note that at one end, 3′ position of sugar is free while at the other end, 5′ position is free, hence they are known as 3′ end and 5′ ends, respectively. This situation is similar to polypeptide chains which have free N-terminal and free C-terminal ends.

Structure of DNA

DNA is the short name of deoxyribonucleic acid. As the name speaks, it contains deoxyribose sugar which is linked to phosphoric acid. The sugar-phosphate forms the backbone of the DNA molecule. The nitrogenous purine bases present are adenine and guanine and pyrimidine bases present are cytosine and thymine. The bases stung out of the sugar phosphate backbone. The molecular weight is very high—about 2 billion

(2×10^9). It may contain 1 million bases arranged in a continuous line.

In fact, there are two polynucleotide chains which are complementary with respect to bases. The two chains are coiled to form a structure similar to double helix or a spiral staircase. The two chains are held together by means of hydrogen bonding between adenine of one chain to thymine of another and guanine of one chain to cytosine of another and *vice versa* (Fig. 11.1). The hydrogen bonding is believed to involve keto and amino groups of the bases. Although the hydrogen bonds are weak bonds, but the combined action of several of them makes the two chains held together very tightly.

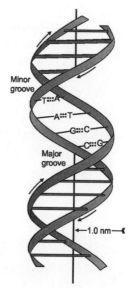

Fig. 11.1: Structure of DNA

Structure of RNA

RNA or ribonucleic acid contains ribose sugar. It has same bases—adenine, guanine, cytosine, but thymine is replaced by its demethylated form uracil. In contrast to DNA, it is a single stranded molecule.

There are various types of RNA molecules, messenger RNA (mRNA), transfer RNA (tRNA) or soluble RNA (sRNA) and ribosomal RNA (rRNA).

mRNA is a linear, single chain molecule. The molecular weight is around 1 million. The polynucleotides are arranged in a continuous line.

sRNA or tRNA is made up of only 73 to 93 nucleotides. A number of them exist. Each binds a different amino acid. It has folded structure which looks like a "clover leaf". One of the ends binds amino acids. Each tRNA has a particular triplet code called "anticodon" which interacts to one of the specific regions of mRNA (Fig. 11.2).

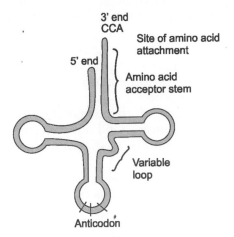

Fig. 11.2: Structure of tRNA

RNA is also found in ribosomes. They are spherical in shape and are attached on rough endoplasmic reticulum. RNA accounts for 60% of their weight, the rest is proteins. A number of proteins and RNA molecules are discovered to be present in the two subunits of ribosomes (Fig. 11.3).

BIOLOGICAL SIGNIFICANCE OF NUCLEIC ACIDS

1. **Choromsomes are nucleoproteins:** Each living cell contains a fixed number of chromosomes in the nucleus. The eukaryotic chromosomes contain DNA and basic proteins (histones). DNA is wrapped around protein to give a product called nucleosome (Fig. 11.4) which is themselves coiled to form chromatin.

The DNA is organized in such a way that each segment acts as a functional unit of heredity called genes. The DNA is

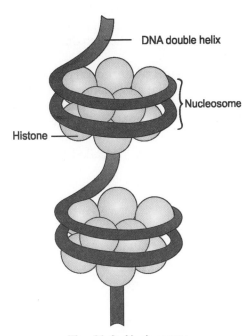

Fig. 11.4: Nucleosome

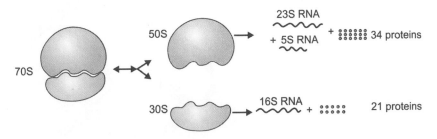

Fig. 11.3: Ribosome and its constituents

highly folded to form the compact structure found in the nucleus of higher organisms.

2. **Cell Division:** The double stranded structure of DNA is of great biological significance in cell division because it permits its own replication. During cell division, the two complementary strands of DNA separate out, each serves as template for the synthesis of its complementary strand by the enzyme, **DNA polymerase**, by directing synthesis of complementary base pairs which can be hydrogen bond (adenine for thymine and *vice versa*, and guanine for cytosine and *vice versa*). As a result, now there are two exactly identical DNA molecules— each one can go to the two daughter cells (Fig. 11.5).

3. **Transmission of hereditary characters:** It is known that all genetic information is coded in the sequence of nucleotides (or bases) in the DNA present in the chromosomes. A functional unit of chromosomal DNA is called a gene. This sequence is same in all the cell's chromosomes and is preserved during cell division and is transferred from parents to offsprings after fertilization of the ovum with the sperm.

4. **Protein synthesis:** DNA and RNA are also involved in the protein synthesis in the cell. The information about the amino acid sequence of the protein to be synthesized is contained in the base sequence of DNA present in the nucleus. In order to transmit this information to protein synthesizing site in the cytoplasm, the DNA molecule first separates into two chains, and then a complementary chain of RNA is synthesized over separated DNA chain to form a hybrid helix (Fig. 11.6). This is accomplished by the enzyme **RNA polymerase** which incorporates ribose as sugar and uracil (and not thymine) as a complementary base to adenine. The whole process is similar to DNA duplication discussed earlier. Finally the RNA chain separates from the hybrid

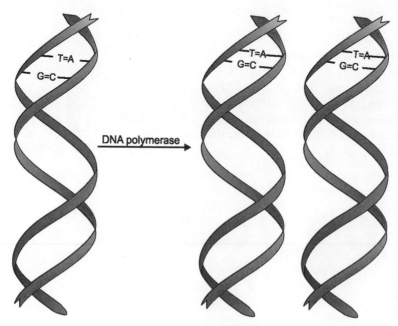

Fig. 11.5: Replication of DNA

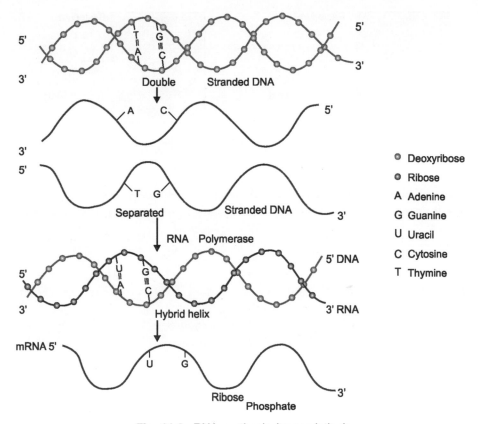

Fig. 11.6: RNA synthesis (transcription)

molecule and move out of nucleus to attach to endoplasmic reticulum. This RNA is called messenger RNA. It takes part in protein synthesis wherein information coded in its base sequence is translated in terms of amino acid sequence of the protein. Protein synthesis is described in detail in chapter on protein metabolism.

5. **Viruses are nucleoproteins:** A virus is either a DNA or RNA nucleoprotein. For example, influenza virus is made of RNA, while adenovirus contains DNA. In order to exist independently and reproduce, a living cell must possess both types of nucleic acids. Thus, viruses which lack one or the other type of nucleic acid must associate with other living cells to provide for their reproduction. A virus is,

therefore, a parasite entity that invades a living cell and alters the metabolism of host cell by directing the synthesis of nucleic acid and protein of which the virus is composed (Fig. 11.7).

6. **Cancer:** There are indications that both the virus and cancer are closely associated. Certain types of neoplasms are believed to be caused by a virus (Burkitt's lymphoma). As the cancer is uncontrolled growth, it has been suggested that there are cancer genes (proto-oncogenes and oncogenes) in everyone but normally they are dormant. Under certain conditions, these are activated with the result that the cancer is manifested. The promoter substance may be anything from a virus to a carcinogen or a hormone.

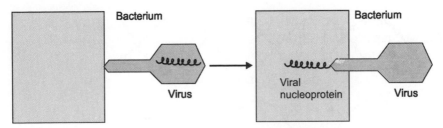

Fig. 11.7: Virus-host cell interaction

7. **Mutation:** The base sequence of DNA genome is very important in determining the characteristics of a person. Any change in a base at any place is called mutation. It would profoundly alter the message contained in DNA. A mutation may be caused by physical agents like radiations or chemical agents, like, acridine dye. The consequence of mutation is formation of altered protein or enzyme molecule which may result in profound effect on overall metabolism in the body. This is the cause of several hereditary diseases called inborn errors (diseases) of metabolism.

8. **Genetic engineering:** Engineering, as we all know is designing, construction and repair of structures of non-living things, so genetic engineering is the construction and repair of the genes of living things. Now it is possible to synthesize a gene in the laboratory and then introduce it into the living cell which will synthesize protein represented by that gene. Researchers have been able to treat diabetes mellitus, sickle cell anemia and thalassemia in animals by this technique. Although it is in its infancy, it holds a bright future for replacing defective genes in humans which are responsible for a variety of ailments.

BIOSYNTHESIS OF PURINES

The synthesis of purine is one of the most complicated pathways, hence, it will not be discussed in detail; instead an outline of

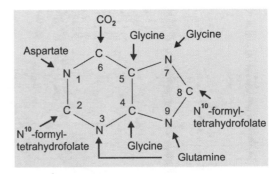

Sources of the individual atoms in the purine ring

synthesis will be given. However, before considering synthesis, it is pertinent to see the sources of different atoms which make up a purine ring.

The atoms of the purine ring are contributed by a number of compounds:

i. Carbon at position 4, 5 and nitrogen at 7 from glycine.

ii. Nitrogen at 1 from aspartic acid.

iii. Nitrogen at 3 and 9 from glutamine.

iv. Carbon at 2 and 8 from formate.

v. Carbon at 6 from respiratory CO_2.

Synthesis: Mammals are capable of synthesizing purine nucleotides and are not dependent on exogenous sources and hence, they are phototrophic. Inosine monophosphate (IMP) is formed first amongst purine nucleosides and then AMP and GMP are formed from it. The purine ring is constructed by a series of reactions that add the donated carbons and nitrogens to a pre-formed ribose-5-phosphate supplied by HMP shunt pathway to finally form purine nucleotide.

Salvage pathway of purine nucleotide synthesis: Purines obtained from normal turnover of cellular nucleic acids or from the diet and not degraded can be converted into nucleoside triphosphates and used by the body. This is referred to as the "**Salvage pathway**" for purines.

A. Adenine phosphoribosyl transferase (APRTase)

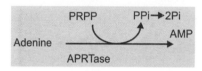

Thus, ribose-5-phosphate is transferred from PRPP to the purine base hypoxanthine to form the nucleotide, IMP (inosine monophosphate).

B. Hypoxanthine–guanine phosphoribosyl transferase (HGPRTase)

Both the enzymes utilize phosphoribosyl (PRPP) as the source of the ribose-5-phosphate group. The release of pyrophosphate and further hydrolysis to inorganic phosphate makes the reaction irreversible. A deficiency of enzyme HGPRT causes the disease called Lesch-Nyhan syndrome.

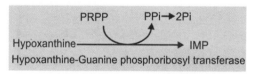

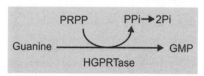

Degradation of purine nucleotides: Purines are catabolized to uric acid. An average of 600–800 mg of uric acid is excreted by human beings in urine. Adenine nucleotide and guanine nucleotide forms a common product, xanthine, which is finally converted to uric acid by the enzyme xanthine oxidase.

AMP → Inosine → Hypoxanthine → Xanthine → Uric acid

GMP → Guanosine → Guanine → Xanthine → Uric acid

Uric acid is excreted in urine. Chronic elevation of uric acid in blood occurs in 3% of the population. The excess uric acid in various fluids results in *Gout* and also results in *arthritic pain* in joints due to deposition in cartilaginous tissue. The big toe is more susceptible. This condition is discussed in detail at the end of this chapter.

SYNTHESIS OF PYRIMIDINES

Before considering the synthesis of pyrimidines, let us look at the sources of atoms in pyrimidine ring.

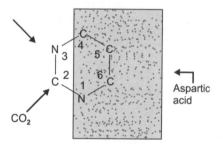

Sources of individual atoms in the pyrimidine ring amide nitrogen of glutamine

The sources of the carbon and nitrogen atoms in pyrimidine ring are:

- N1, C4, C5 and C6 from aspartic acid
- C2 from CO_2
- N3 from glutamine

In order to avoid complexity only, outline of pyrimidine synthesis will be described.

While purine synthesis takes place on preexisting ribose-5'-phosphate, the pyrimidine ring is synthesized before being attached to ribose-5'-phosphate which is donated by PRPP.

The first step is the synthesis of carbamoyl phosphate from glutamine and CO_2 in the cytosol. This reaction is comparable to first reaction of urea cycle which occurs in mitochondria and uses ammonia and CO_2.

It may be noted that both purine and pyrimidine synthesis require glutamine and PRPP as essential precursors.

Catabolism of pyrimidines: While purine ring is not cleaved in humans, the pyrimidine ring is opened and degraded to β-alanine and β-aminoisobutyrate, which thus form acetyl CoA and succinyl CoA, respectively on further breakdown.

Salvage pathway: Pyrimidines obtained from the diet or by tissue degradation can be salvaged and converted into nucleotides by the enzyme pyrimidine phosphoribosyl transferase, which utilizes PRPP as the source of ribose-phosphate. This reaction is similar to purine salvage pathway.

Inborn errors of nucleic acid metabolism: One of the most important metabolic diseases belonging to the purine metabolism is gout.

Gout: Gout is characterized by hyperuricemia and is accompanied by deposition of urate in joints causing joint enlargement, large soft tissue tophi, inflammation, pain and arthritis (Figs 11.8 and 11.9).

Glucose-6-phosphatase deficient persons sometimes develop gout because due to this deficiency, more of glucose-6-phosphate is shunted to HMP shunt pathway resulting into more ribose-5'-phosphate and then more PRPP which form more purine nucleotides. The catabolism of excessive purines leads to overproduction of uric acid (primary gout, hyperuricemia). Secondary gout may be caused by cancer due to excessive catabolism of nucleic acids leading to hyperuricemia and in renal failure due to impaired elimination of uric acid.

The treatment of gout is by giving drug of choice allopurinol which inhibits xanthine oxidase, resulting into an accumulation of hypoxanthine and xanthine compounds which are more soluble than uric acid. A diet deficient in flesh (food, fish) should be given.

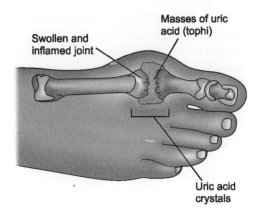

Fig. 11.8: Foot of the patient affected by gout

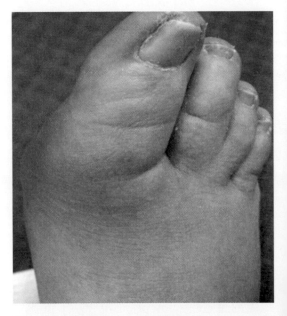

Fig. 11.9: Acute gout with erythema (redness) of the great toe joint

Hypoxanthine →(XO) Xanthine →(XO) Uric acid

Allopurinol

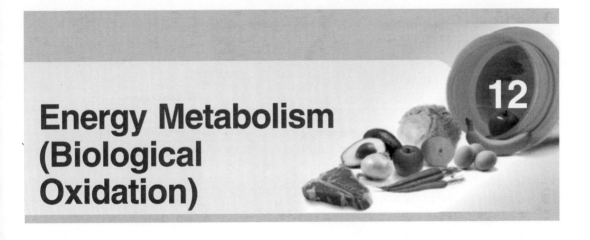

Energy Metabolism (Biological Oxidation)

12

INTRODUCTION

Energy is essential for every living cell and organism to grow, to perform work and to stay alive. Some energy requiring biological processes which involve different types of energy are given below:

Chemical work: Synthesis of nucleic acids and proteins.

Mechanical work: Muscular movement.

Osmotic work: Transport of various salts against concentration gradient.

Electrical work: Electrical impulses in nervous system and brain.

Thermal work: Maintenance of temperature of warm blooded animals.

As we all know that the ultimate source of energy is sunlight which is converted into chemical energy by photosynthesis in plant cells. That chemical energy is utilized by animals by taking it from plants in the form of food. It is again converted into the different form of energy as mentioned above.

Therefore, to understand different life processes, it is very essential to study the quantitative conversion of energy into various forms by applying the rules of thermodynamics into biological systems which is called as "Bioenergetics". In simple words, it is the study of energy in relation to living organisms.

"Energy metabolism is the quantitative study of energy transformations that occur in living cells in relation to the nature and role of various chemical processes responsible for this transformation".

OXIDATION–REDUCTION REACTIONS

All reactions in which addition of oxygen or removal of hydrogen or electrons are involved are called oxidation reactions and removal of oxygen or addition of hydrogen or electrons called as reduction reactions. Oxidation and reduction reactions are coupled reactions as shown in Table 12.1.

Oxidation–reduction reactions are coupled reactions. They depend on redox potential. A compound having more positive (+) redox potential will oxidize and more negative (–) will reduce.

$$AH_2 + B \longrightarrow BH_2 + A$$

The oxidation–reduction reactions in biological systems are catalyzed by enzymes which are given below:

Enzymes of Oxidation-Reduction Reactions

1. **Oxidases:** The hydrogen or reducing equivalents transfer directly to molecular O_2 to form water, e.g. cytochrome oxidase.

2. **Dehydrogenases:** They catalyze transfer of hydrogen from one substrate to another or to oxygen. Many dehydrogenases use coenzymes of vitamin niacin or riboflavin.

Table 12.1: Oxidation and reduction

Oxidation	Reduction
1. Addition of oxygen	1. Removal of oxygen
$RCH_2OH \xrightarrow[O_2 \quad H_2O]{} RCOOH$	$H_2O \longrightarrow \frac{1}{2}O_2 + 2H^+ + 2e^\ominus$
2. Removal of hydrogen	2. Addition of hydrogen
$RCH_2OH \xrightarrow[2H]{Dehydrogenase} RCHD$	$NAD^+ + 2H^+ + 2e^\ominus \longrightarrow NADH + H^+$
3. Removal of electrons	3. Addition of electrons
$Fe^{2+} \xrightarrow{e^-} Fe^{3+}$	$2H^+ + 2e^- \longrightarrow H_2$

$$AH_2 + FAD \quad\quad A + FADH_2$$
$$FADH_2 + O_2 \quad\quad FAD + H_2O_2$$

3. Hydroperoxidases: Catalyze reduction of H_2O_2 to H_2O with liberation of oxygen. They are of two types:

  a. Peroxidase: Transfer of oxygen of H_2O_2 to a substrate forming water. Example: Thyroidal iodine peroxidase.

$$H_2O_2 + AH_2 \rightarrow A + 2H_2O$$
$$1^\ominus + H_2O_2 \xrightarrow{Peroxidase} IO^- + H_2O$$

  b. Catalase: Uses hydrogen peroxide as electron donor as well as electron acceptor. For example, catalase specifically catalyze break down of H_2O_2 to water and oxygen.

$$2H_2O_2 \longrightarrow 2H_2O + O_2$$

4. Oxygenases: They incorporate O_2 directly into their substrate but are not concerned with energy production.

  a. Dioxygenases: Catalyze incorporation of both the atoms of O_2 into substrate. Example: Carotene dioxygenase.

$$A + O_2 \rightarrow AO_2$$

  b. Monooxygenases or hydroxylases: Incorporate one atom of O_2 into substrate to form a hydroxyl group while other oxygen atom is reduced. Example: Phenylalanine hydroxylase.

$$O_2 + \text{Phenylalanine} + \text{Tetrahydrobiopterin} \rightarrow$$
$$\text{Tyrosine} + \text{Dihydrobiopterin} + H_2O$$

BIOLOGICAL OXIDATION

The energy rich compounds undergo a series of metabolic reactions and finally get oxidized to CO_2 and H_2O. The simple reaction of oxidation of glucose is given below:

$$C_6H_{12}O_6 + 6O_2 \longrightarrow 6CO_2 + 6H_2O + \text{Energy}$$

All the three energy rich nutrients release energy as indicated in Fig. 12.1

The energy liberated in these processes goes to two main fates—some part is converted into heat and the rest is trapped as chemical energy in the form of ATP in mitochondria.

ELECTRON TRANSPORT CHAIN

The reducing equivalents from various metabolic intermediates are transferred to coenzyme NAD^+ and FAD to produce NADH and $FADH_2$, respectively. These compounds get oxidized by transferring there electrons to oxygen. This is not a direct process, a lot of intermediates are involved in this in the form of a sequence or chain called as electron transport chain (ETC),

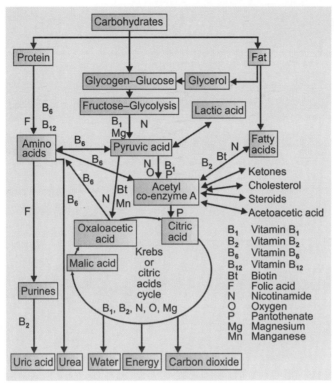

Fig. 12.1: Energy rich nutrients and their breakdown to liberate energy

which is also called respiratory chain (Fig. 12.2). It occurs in inner wall of mitochondria.

The mitochondrion is the main site for energy production in cell. That is why, it is also called power house of the cell. Inner mitochondrial membrane is a highly folded and specialized structure. It is rich in proteins and enzymes and impermeable to ions like Na^+, K^+, H^+ and small molecules like ATP and ADP. Inner side of inner mitochondrial wall contains specialized particles (F_0F_1 particles) which are the sites for oxidative phosphorylation (Fig. 12.3).

Components of ETC

1. **Nicotinamide nucleotides:** It is produced in the body from vitamin niacin. NAD^+ is more actively involved in ETC. It is reduced to NADH + H^+ by dehydrogenases with the removal of two hydrogen atoms from the substrate.

2. **Flavoproteins:** These are the enzymes that catalyze the oxidation–reduction reactions using either FMN or FAD as a co-factor which is derived from vitamin riboflavin.

3. **Ubiquinone:** It is also called as coenzyme Q. It is a lipophillic electron carrier and accepts electrons from $FMNH_2$ produced outside ETC. It is freely diffusible within the lipid bilayer of the inner mitochondrial membrane.

4. **Cytochromes:** These are iron containing electron transfer proteins of inner mitochondrial membrane. Mainly five types of cytochromes are known which participate in electron transfer in ETC. These are Cyt b, c_1, c, a, a_3.

The cytochrome oxidase is the terminal component of ETC which can directly react with molecular O_2. It is the complex of Cyt aa_3.

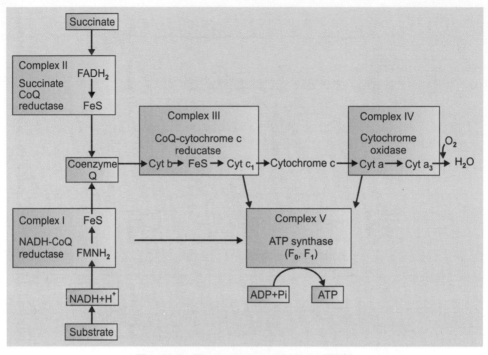

Fig. 12.2: Electron transport chain (ETC)

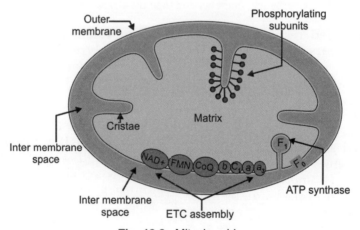

Fig. 12.3: Mitochondria

5. **Iron–Sulphur proteins:** These proteins contain one iron co-ordinately linked to four sulphur of cysteine amino acid of protein. It participates in one electron transfer.

The different components described above form complexes of respiratory chain which in turn transfer electrons from one complex to another according to their redox potential. The compounds having more positive redox potential will accept electrons due to the higher affinity for them. The complexes of respiratory chain as indicated in Fig. 12.2 are described in detail further.

Complexes of ETC

There are five complexes as discussed below.

1. **Complex I: Electron transfer from NADH to ubiquinone:** This is present in inner mitochondrial membrane and also called as NADH dehydrogenase. It accepts a proton from water in the matrix. The enzyme complex first transfers a reducing equivalent from NADH to FMN and then to Fe-S protein which in turn transfers it to coenzyme Q.

2. **Complex II: Succinate to ubiquinone:** It is also called as succinate dehydrogenase and it is the only membrane bound enzyme in TCA cycle. Electron transfer takes place from succinate to FAD and from FAD to Fe-S proteins and finally transfers to coenzyme Q.

3. **Complex III: Ubiquinone to cytochrome c:** This complex is also known as cytochrome bc_1 complex or ubiquinone–cytochrome c oxido-reductase. Electrons are transferred from cyt b to Fe-S protein and from Fe-S protein to cyt c_1 and from cyt c_1 to cyt c from where electrons are transferred to next complex.

4. **Complex IV: Cytochrome oxidase:** Reduction of O_2 is the main event here. This complex contains cyt a and cyt a_3. Complex IV causes net movement of protons from matrix to inter membrane space and in cytochrome oxidase reaction, four electrons are transferred from four cyt c molecules and four hydrogen ions are transferred to oxygen to form two molecules of water.

5. **Complex V:** It consists of ATP synthase and present in inner mitochondrial membrane. It is the main site for oxidative phosphorylation.

OXIDATIVE PHOSPHORYLATION

It is the phosphorylation of ADP to ATP using energy from proton pump fuelled by electron transport chain.

$$ADP + Pi \xrightarrow[\text{Energy from ETC}]{} ATP \text{ (energy trapped in P-P bond)}$$

This is the major process by which aerobic organisms obtain their energy from food.

The ATP generating sites in ETC are:

i. NAD-CoQ reductase (between FMN $\rightarrow$ FeS)
ii. Co-Q Cytochrome c reductase (between Cyt b $\rightarrow$ Cyt c_1)
iii. Cytochrome oxidase (between cyt a_3 $\rightarrow$ O_2)

About 42% of released energy is trapped as high energy bonds of ATP. The energy released at each step is proportional to difference in redox potential.

Mechanism of oxidative phosphorylation: Redox potential is intimately related to free energy change. Energy released is proportional to potential difference. The electrons are transferred from agents with more negative to less negative potential. The energy is released in the form of packets which is trapped in high energy phosphate bonds of ATP, known as oxidative phosphorylation.

Several theories have been put forward to explain ATP generation during electron transport. The chemiosmotic theory is now universally accepted.

Chemiosmotic theory: According to this theory, the transport of electrons in the electron transport chain causes pumping out of protons across the inner mitochondrial membrane into the inter membrane space (Fig. 12.3) to create a proton (H^+) gradient. The accompanying membrane potential is of the order of –0.15 V, the matrix being negative. Simultaneously, the inner compartment becomes alkaline and the outer compartment more acidic. It is conjectured that a pH gradient of 0.05 units across the inner mitochondrial membrane is created.

The proton gradient is the immediate driving force of the phosphorylation of ADP which proceeds through enzyme F_1-ATPase in the inner membrane, more correctly known as ATP synthase. It is made up of several polypeptides.

Uncouplers: Some lipid soluble weak acids such as 2,4-dinitrophenol (DNP) uncouple oxidative phosphorylation. Uncouplers reduce or nullify the proton gradient; consequently they inhibit the synthesis of ATP by ATP synthase. They may simultaneously promote the ATPase activity of the F_1 unit by enhancing the H^+ concentration in the matrix. The energy released is dissipated as heat. Thyroxine hormone is also such a substance which regulates energy production in the body. Both thyroxine and 2,4-dinitrophenol are used as drugs to reduce body weight on account of their ability to release nutrient energy as heat which is then dissipated.

The cold blooded animals have brown adipose tissue in back and neck which are rich in electron carriers and can carry electron transport (oxidation) uncoupled to phosphorylation with the result that much heat is released to protect from surrounding cold.

Inhibitors: Many compounds inhibit oxidative phosphorylation. For example, cyanide and carbon monoxide inhibit cytochrome oxidase system. They act as strong poisons because they block cellular respiration or electron transport chain (ETC).

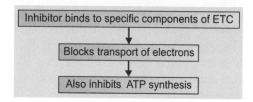

There are several well-known drugs and toxins that inhibit oxidative phosphorylation (Table 12.2). Although any one of these toxins inhibits only one enzyme in the electron transport chain, inhibition of any step in this process will halt the rest of the process. For example, if oligomycin inhibits ATP synthase, protons cannot pass back into the mitochondrion. As a result, the proton pumps are unable to operate, as the gradient becomes too strong for them to overcome. NADH is then no longer oxidized and the citric acid cycle ceases to operate because the concentration of NAD^+ falls below the concentration that these enzymes can use.

Table 12.2: Drugs and toxins which inhibit oxidative phosphorylation

Compounds	Used as	Effects on oxidative phosphorylation
Cyanide Carbon dioxide Azide	Poisons Poisons Poisons	Inhibits the electron transport chain by binding more strongly than oxygen to the Fe-Cu centre in cytochrome c oxidase, preventing the reduction of oxygen.
Oligomycin	Antibiotic	Inhibits ATP synthase by blocking the flow of protons through the F_0 subunits.
CCCP 2,4-Dinitrophenol	Poisons Poisons	Ionophores that disrupt the proton gradient by carrying protons across a membrane. This ionophore uncouples proton pumping from ATP synthesis because it carries protons across the inner mitochondrial membrane.
Rotenone	Pesticide	Prevents the transfer of electrons from complex I to ubiquinone by blocking the ubiquinone binding site.
Malonate Oxaloacetate	Inhibitor Inhibitor	Competitive inhibitors of succinate dehydrogenase (complex II)

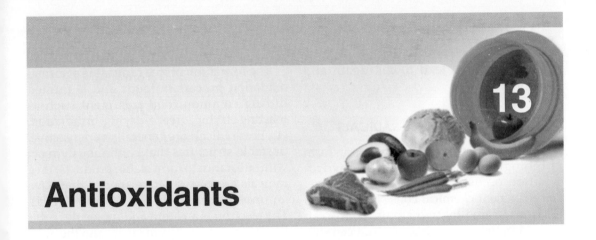

Antioxidants

13

INTRODUCTION

Antioxidants are the compounds that scavenge free radicals and help in protecting the body from a load of free radicals which are generated in metabolic processes every day. They are any substances that prevent cell destruction by free radicals. The free radicals are charged particles found in the environment and also produced by chemical processes in the body. The antioxidants combine with free radicals and neutralize their damaging effects (Fig. 13.1).

FREE RADICALS

Chemically, the free radicals are atoms or molecules with an unpaired electron and which are generally very reactive. They are produced continuously in cells either as accidental byproducts of metabolism or deliberately during, for example, phagocytosis. The most important reactants in free radical biochemistry in aerobic cells are oxygen and its radical derivatives (superoxide and hydroxyl radical), hydrogen peroxide and transition metals. Cells have developed a comprehenzive array of antioxidant defenses to prevent free radical formation or limit their damaging effects. These include enzymes to decompose peroxides, proteins to sequester transition metals and a range of compounds to 'scavenge' free radicals. Reactive free radicals formed within cells can oxidize

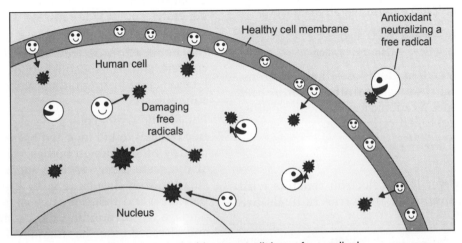

Fig. 13.1: Antioxidant neutralizing a free radical

biomolecules and lead to cell death and tissue injury.

FORMATION OF FREE RADICALS

Dehydrogenation is the most common form of biological oxidation. Most dehydrogenation occurs by C–H bond cleavage. Since covalent chemical consists of pairs of electrons shared by two atoms, bonds can cleaved in two ways—one electron can stay with one atom or each atom. In most reactions, both electron stays with each atom. Cleavage of C–H bond always produces two ions (Fig. 13.2).

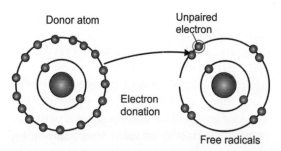

Fig. 13.2: Free radical formation by unpaired election

1. If the carbon retains both electrons, carbon containing compound becomes a carbanion (i.e. with negative charge).

$$R\text{–}C\text{–}H \longrightarrow R = C: + H^+$$
Carbanion   proton

2. If the carbon atom loses both electrons, the carbon containing compound becomes a cationic ion (i.e. with positive charge) called carbocation.

$$R\text{–}C\text{–}H^- \longrightarrow R\text{–}C^+: + H^-:$$
Carbocation   hydride ion

However if one electron remains with each compound, then free radicals are formed.

$$R_1 O\text{–}OR_2 \longrightarrow R_1 O' + {}'OR_2$$

The formation of free radicals is a normal oxidation process in foods and is formed during common food treatment such as toasting, frying, freeze drying, irradiation, etc. Free radicals are generally very reactive, unstable structures that continuously react with substance to form stable products. Free radicals are very reactive species that have an unpaired electron, e.g. hydroxyl (OH). The electron is an atom and molecules orbit the nucleus in shells and layers and the most stable configuration occurs when these electrons are in pairs that orbit in opposite directions. If an atom or molecule within the body loses or gain an electron, the resulting entity is always reactive and can react and damage DNA, proteins, lipids or carbohydrates. Cellular damage caused by oxygen free radicals species cause cancer, atherosclerosis, cataract and retinopathy. All the degenerative diseases in old people may be due to the cumulative effects of free radicals damage.

Processes that Generate Free Radicals

Some of the processes that generate free radicals include:

- Electrons transport chain—free radicals are byproducts of the electron transport chain.

- Dissolution of oxygen hemoglobin generates superoxide radicals.

- Certain environmental factors increase the generation of free radicals, e.g. cigarette smoke, exposure to high oxygen tension and ionizing radiation including sunlight.

- Phagocytic white cells generate oxygen free radicals to kill ingested bacteria and destroy other 'foreign bodies'. They can also secrete these reactive species into surrounding tissues (e.g. to kill large parasites) and this can cause significant damage to surrounding tissues. Injured and diseased tissue has high level of free radicals.

Role of Oxygen Free Radicals

The oxygen free radicals can react with DNA to cause break in DNA chain and alteration of bases (mutation). This could initiate carcinogenesis. Free radicals can peroxidize polyunsaturated fatty acids (PUFA) residue in low density lipoprotein (LDL). This oxidized LDL is taken up by macrophages and generates foam cells and this ultimately leads to scarring and fibrosis of artery walls seen in atherosclerosis. Unoxidized LDL is considered relatively benign in its effects upon artery wall. The reaction of free radicals involves the loss and gain of electrons and this creates another free radical, which initiate damaging chain reaction unless a free radical's activity is suppressed by antioxidant. For example, peroxidation of a PUFA will generate another stable compound (the lipid peroxyl radical) and this reacts with another fatty acid to produce stable lipid peroxides (Fig. 13.3). Susceptibility of PUFA to free radicals damage is one of the concerns about recommending high level of PUFA in a diet.

ANTIOXIDANTS

The antioxidants are those entities which neutralize free radicals and limit their tissue damaging effects. The primary enzymatic defense includes superoxide dismutase, catalase, peroxidase, etc. Non-enzymatic defense includes glutathione, ascorbate, beta carotene, flavonoid and phenolic acids (Fig. 13.4).

Mechanisms Involved in the Disposal of Free Radicals by Antioxidants

- Superoxide dismutase (Zn containing) converts superoxide radicals to H_2O_2.

$$O_2^- + O_2^- + 2H^+ \xrightarrow{\text{SOD}} H_2O_2 + O_2$$

- Glutathione peroxidase (Se containing) converts H_2O_2 to water.

$$H_2O_2 + \text{reduced glutathione} \xrightarrow{\text{Glutathione peroxidase}}$$
$$H_2O + \text{oxidized glutathione}$$

- Glutathione reductase (B_2 containing) regenerates glutathione.

$$\text{Oxidized glutathione} \xrightarrow{\text{Glutathione reductase}} \text{Reduced glutathione}$$

- The enzyme catalase (Fe containing) converts H_2O_2 into water and O_2.

$$2H_2O_2 \xrightarrow{\text{Catalase}} 2H_2O + O_2$$

- Vitamin E can quench free radicals when it is oxidized.

$$\text{Free radicals} + \text{Vitamin E} \longrightarrow \text{Water} + \text{oxidized vitamin E}$$

$$\text{Lipid peroxyl radical} + \text{Vitamin E} \longrightarrow \text{Stable hydroperoxide} + \text{Oxidized vitamin E}$$

- Vitamin E can be regenerated by a mechanism that involves vitamin C.

$$\text{Oxidized vitamin E} \xrightarrow{\text{Vitamin C}} \text{Vitamin E}$$

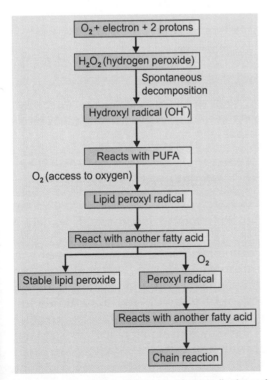

Fig. 13.3: Formation of hydroxyl free radicals and its role in lipid peroxidation

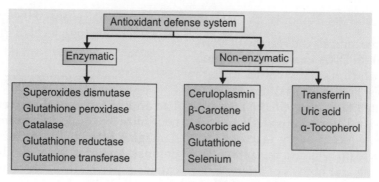

Fig. 13.4: Antioxidant defense system

FREE RADICALS IN CAUSING DISEASES

The free radicals have been implicated in the etiology of the host of degenerative diseases including cardiovascular diseases, diabetes, cancer, Alzheimer's diseases, retinal degeneration, ischemic dementia and other neurodegenerative disorders and aging. In addition, they also play a role not only in acute condition, such as trauma, stroke and infection, but also in physical exercise and stress.

Cardiovascular Diseases

A high fat diet tends to raise the LDL cholesterol concentration and further cigarette smoking increases free radical production. If the diet does not provide adequate antioxidant protection then scavenging the free radical becomes problem.

The free radicals might contribute to the risk of cardiovascular diseases as shown in Fig. 13.5.

Ageing

An increasing number of diseases and disorders as well as ageing process itself, demonstrate link either directly and indirectly to these reactive and potentially destructive molecules. Reduction of free radicals or decreasing their rate of production may delay ageing and onset of degenerative condition associated with ageing.

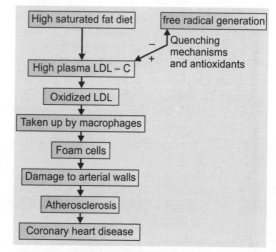

Fig. 13.5: Hypothesis showing how free radicals might contribute to the risk of cardiovascular disease

NATURAL AND DIET-DERIVED ANTIOXIDANTS

Our daily foods contain a wide variety of free radical scavenging molecules. Vegetables, fruits, tea and wine are the products rich in natural oxidant compounds. Fruits and vegetables are rich source of antioxidants, flavonoids and vitamins. One can get sufficient quantities of these by consuming at least 4–5 servings of fruits and vegetables daily.

The dietary antioxidants may contribute to the decrease of cardiovascular diseases by reduction of free radicals formation as well as oxidative damage by protection of LDL oxidation platelets aggregation and inhibiting synthesis of pro-inflammatory cytokines. Epidemiological studies have shown that a higher intake of these compounds is also associated with a lower risk of mortality from cancer and coronary heart diseases.

Some of the substances in food that are known to have an antioxidant effect are:

- The essential minerals—selenium (rice and wheat), zinc.
- Vitamin C (found in high abundance in many fruits and vegetables and is also found in cereals, beef, poultry and fish) and vitamin E (wheat germ, safflower, corn and soybean oils, and also found in mangoes, nuts, broccoli and other foods).
- β-carotene and several other carotenoids including lycopene (abundant in tomatoes), lutein and zeaxanthin (found in green leafy vegetables), α-carotene (carrots, tomatoes, green beans) and cryptoxanthin (papaya, oranges, corn and watermelon), and other plant pigments, such as polyphenols found in some fruits, tea, olive oil and red wine and the flavonoid found in grapes, nuts, oranges and strawberries.

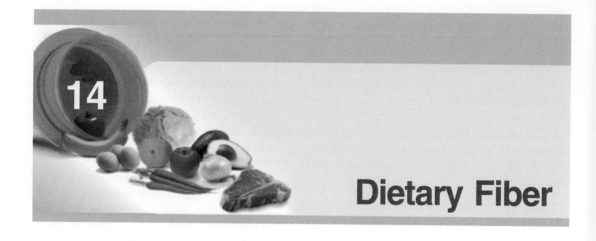

Dietary Fiber

14

INTRODUCTION

The dietary fiber is defined as that part of plant material in our diet which is resistant to digestion. This term includes all indigestible polysaccharides, lignin, pectins, gums and mucilage (flax seeds), cellulose, hemicellulose, and even bacterial degradation products of undigestible polysaccharides. Dietary fiber is thus not limited to the substances which can be recovered in feces but also chemically inert substances. Table 14.1 gives fiber content of various food items—fruits, vegetables and cereals.

TYPES OF FIBER

1. **Cellulose:** It is the well known component of fiber, consisting of 3000 or more glucose molecules linked together in long chains by β-1, 4 bonds to form elastic walls of plant cells. It swells in water. It is found in bran, legumes, peas, root vegetables, the cabbage family, the outer covering of seeds and most fruits.

2. **Hemicelluloses:** They are branched polymers not related to cellulose and are not cellulose precursors as was formerly presumed. They contain mostly xylose, some galactose, mannose, arabinose and other sugars. Hemicellulose is a major constituent of cereal fiber, found in bran and whole grains.

3. **Lignin:** It is present in the cell wall, made of phenyl propane units and is not digestible. This is the primary non-carbohydrate component of fiber. It is highest in mature root vegetables like carrots or fruits with edible seeds like strawberries.

4. **Polyfructoses:** Examples are inulins and oligofructans, found in onions, garlic, artichokes and soya bean.

5. **Gums:** These are substances secreted by a plant at injury sites. They are composed of various sugars and sugar derivatives. Found in oatmeal, barley and legumes.

6. **Mucilage:** Gelatinous substances found in most plants.

7. **Pectins:** Water-soluble and gel-forming substances found in apples, strawberries and citrus fruits.

8. **Resistant starches:** These are starches classified as fibers because they are not digested by the body. They are found in whole legumes, potatoes and bananas and plantains.

The physiological role of dietary fiber in human nutrition was so far believed to be related to 'crude fiber' which helped the bowel movement. The components of dietary fiber are important in influencing such physiological properties as fecal bulking, retention of water in the stool or binding bile salt.

FUNCTIONS OF FIBER

- **Regular bowel movements:** The fiber is the edible part of fruits, vegetables and

Table 14.1: Fiber content of food

Total dietary fiber (%)		Total dietary fiber (%)	
Fruits			
Apple	1.42	Peas	7.75
Banana	2.6		
Cherry	1.24		
Grapefruit	0.44	**Root vegetables**	
Orange	1.90	Carrot	2.90
Peach	2.28		
Pear	2.44	Potato	3.41
Plum	1.52		
Strawberry	2.12		
Tomato	1.40	**Cereals**	
Leafy vegetables		Whole wheat flour	13.51
Broccoli top	3.60	Bran, sieved	30.60
Brussels sprout	4.22	Bran, coarse	48.00
Cabbage	3.44	Oatmeal	7.66
Onion	1.30	Rice	2.74

grains that the body cannot digest. Since they are not absorbed into the body, dietary fibers are not considered a nutrient. Some fiber dissolves easily in water and becomes soft in the intestines, while insoluble fiber passes almost unchanged through the intestines. Both kinds of fiber are required to make stools soft and easy to pass. Fiber also prevents constipation, which makes it easy for bowel muscles to move even hard stool. The lack of fiber is believed to be the main cause of increased pressure in the colon that may cause the weak colon spots to bulge out and become diverticula.

- **Reducing blood cholesterol levels:** Viscous fibers lower cholesterol levels by reducing the absorption of dietary cholesterol. In addition, they combine with bile acids which are removed from circulation and do not make it back to the liver. As a result, the liver must use additional cholesterol to manufacture new bile acids. Soluble fiber may also reduce the amount of cholesterol synthesized by the liver.

- **Normalizing blood sugar levels:** Viscous fibers are also involved in controlling blood glucose levels because they slow down the rate at which food leaves the stomach and delay the absorption of glucose after a meal. Viscous fibers also increase insulin sensitivity. As a result, viscous fibers are believed to play a role in the prevention and treatment of type 2 diabetes mellitus.

- **Supporting bowel regularity:** Fermentable fibers are fermented by the intestinal flora, the bacteria and fungi that live in the intestines. The fermentation of dietary fiber in the large intestine produces a short-chain fatty acid, butyric acid, which is used as fuel by the cells of the large intestine and helps maintain the health of the colon. Fermentable fibers also help maintain healthy populations of bacteria in the intestinal flora. Fibers that are not fermentable help maintain bowel regularity by increasing the bulk of the feces and decreasing the time required by fecal matter to move through the intestines.

BENEFITS OF DIETARY FIBER

There are several epidemiological studies suggesting an association between fiber intake and obesity or coronary heart disease. Dietary fiber can modulate body weight by various mechanisms. Fiber-rich foods usually have lower energy content, which contributes to a decrease into the energy supplied by the diet. Foods rich in fiber need to be chewed longer, leading to an increase in the time needed to eat the food and in the feeling of satiety. The fibers which make up viscous solutions also delay the passage of food from the stomach to duodenum and contribute to an increase in satiety and a decrease in energy consumption. In the intestine, the incorporation of fiber may complicate the union between digestive enzymes and their substrate, thus slowing down the absorption of nutrients. It is also important to note that the effects of dietary fiber consumption on body weight may be related to different gut hormones which regulate satiety, energy intake and/or pancreatic functions.

A variety of diseases in fiber deficient diet includes appendicitis, constipation, diverticular diseases of the colon, polyps and cancer of the large bowel, ulcerative colitis, Crohn's disease, varicose veins, deep vein thrombosis, piles, hiatus hernia, gall stones, cholecystitis, heart diseases, diabetes, obesity, dental caries, periodontal disease, duodenal ulcer and possibly many other diseases.

a. **In constipation:** The important physiologic effect of fiber is to increase the bulk and retain water content of the stool. The capacity of fiber to increase the bulk of stool varies like 50 g of bran, 100 g raw carrot, 150 g apple or 200 g orange holds 200 ml of water. The transit time is assumed to decrease with low fiber and increase with high fiber diet. Bran has the greatest laxative effects.

b. **In diverticular diseases:** The diverticulosis is a condition characterized by small pouches (diverticula) that form and push outward through weak spots in the large intestine. Once diverticula have formed, there is no way to reverse the process. When diverticula become infected, the condition is called diverticulitis. Most people with diverticulosis do not experience symptoms. As for diverticulitis, the most common symptom is abdominal pain with tenderness around the left side of the lower abdomen. Fever, nausea, vomiting, chills, cramping, and constipation may occur as well. A low-fiber diet is believed to be the main cause of the disease.

It has been shown that increasing the amount of fiber in the diet may reduce symptoms of diverticular disease. The American Dietetic Association recommends a daily intake of 20–35 grams of fiber. A diverticular disease diet will accordingly seek to increase dietary fiber to these levels to prevent constipation and the undue colon pressure that causes diverticula.

c. **In colonic cancer:** A high fiber diet presumed to protect against colonic cancer by decreasing the transit time so allowing less time for the colonic bacteria to produce carcinogen. It has been pointed out that the evidence of colonic cancer throughout the world correlates best with a high intake of dietary fat and protein together with other indices of affluence but poorly, with fiber intake. The overall effect of dietary fiber is related to the type of fecal bulk, colonic microflora, fecal pH, transit time, alteration of nutrient absorption and the postprandial hormone secretion.

d. **In diabetes mellitus:** An increased intake of dietary fiber appears to be useful for the treatment of both obesity and diabetes mellitus. Fiber-rich food is usually satisfying without being calorically dense. Supplementing a normal diet with gel-forming fibers, such as guar gum, leads to an increased satiation probably due to a slower gastric emptying. Recent long-term studies have confirmed the usefulness of viscous fibers as an adjunct to regular dietary treatment of obesity. Apart from a beneficial effect during caloric restriction, dietary fiber may improve some of the metabolic aberrations seen in obesity. Gel-forming fibers are particularly effective in reducing elevated LDL-cholesterol without changing the HDL-fraction. Impaired glucose tolerance or manifest diabetes is also improved. These effects are probably in part associated with the gelling property of the fiber which leads to an increased viscosity of the unstirred layer thereby delaying the absorption process. Other sources of dietary fiber with a high content of viscous gums, such as oats, have been shown to reduce LDL-cholesterol. Increased intake of viscous fiber leads to a gradual reduction in fasting glucose levels in diabetics.

In biliary diseases: For human, adding cellulose to the diet increases fecal bile salts excretion, which may be helpful in biliary diseases.

e. **Irritable bowel syndrome:** The irritable bowel syndrome is treated with a high fiber diet. Perhaps benefit is associated with relief obtained in a constipated patient.

f. **Dental caries:** The damaging effect on teeth with a frequent intake of refined carbohydrate as sugar is well recognized. A high fiber diet usually reduces refined sugar intake and has a beneficial effect on dental caries. Fiber also requires more mastication that promotes salivary flow.

SIDE EFFECTS OF HIGH FIBER DIET

A high fiber diet produces abdominal distention, pain, flatulence and diarrhea and with a high phytate content decreases the absorption of calcium, zinc and iron. This may predispose to osteomalacia and iron deficiency anemia. Decreased zinc absorption in children produces stunted growth and retarded sexual development. In patient with narrowing of the intestinal lumen due to tuberculosis, Crohn's disease or cancer, fibrous foods may produce intestinal obstruction.

When increasing the fiber content of the diet, it is recommended to add fiber progressively, adding just a few grams at a time to allow the intestinal tract to adjust. Otherwise abdominal cramps, gas, bloating and diarrhea or constipation may result. Intake of dietary fiber exceeding of 50 g per day may also lead to intestinal obstruction. Excessive intake of fiber can also cause a fluid imbalance, leading to dehydration, this is why, people who start increasing their fiber intake are often advised to also increase their water intake. Excessive intake of dietary fiber has been linked with reduced absorption of vitamins, minerals, proteins and calories. However, it is unlikely that healthy people who consume fiber in amounts within the recommended ranges will have problems with nutrient absorption.

The parents are urged to use caution when adding extra fiber to their child's diet. Excessive amounts of high-fiber foods may cause a child to fill up quickly, reducing appetite and possibly depriving the child of needed nutrients from a well-balanced diet. Elderly people and those who have had gastrointestinal surgery should also exercise caution when increasing their dietary fiber intake.

Summary of Dietary Fiber

1. The unavailable or indigestible carbohydrate in the diet is called dietary fiber.
2. Dietary fiber is necessary to maintain the normal motility of gastrointestinal tract. The diet rich in fiber improves bowel motility, prevents constipation, decreases

reabsorption of bile acids, thus, lowering cholesterol level and improves glucose tolerance.

3. The most important fibers, their chemical nature and physiological effects are given in Table 14.2.

Table 14.2: Main dietary fibers

Fibers	Chemical nature	Physiological effects
Cellulose	Polymer of glucose	Retains water in feces; promotes peristalsis, increases bowel action
Hemicellulose	Pentoses, hexoses and uronic acid	Retains water in feces, increases bile acid excretion
Pectins	Partially esterified rhamnogalacturans	Absorbs water, slows gastric emptying, binds bile acids and increases their excretion

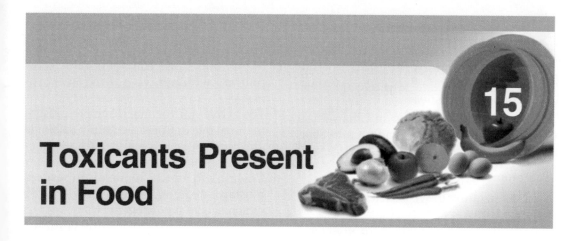

Toxicants Present in Food

INTRODUCTION

The food contains not only the nutrients we need (e.g. carbohydrates, proteins, fats, vitamins and inorganic elements) but also a large number of chemicals, some of which are toxic. Some toxic chemicals may enter the food supply by fortuitous natural mechanisms. These may be of microbial origin and may be environmental pollutants including heavy metals. Chemicals sprayed into plants in the form of pesticides may be present in food of plant origin and may be transmitted through feed grains to animals. There are also substances added to foods for functional purposes, such as preservatives, antioxidants and calorie reduction agents. Toxic compounds are naturally occurring in some plant and animal foods or foods may be contaminated by toxicants during storage. These toxicants cause serious illness in man and some may lead to even death.

The toxicants can be divided into three classes:

a. Naturally occurring toxicants

b. Toxicants from pathogenic micro-organisms

c. Contamination of food with toxic chemicals, pesticides and insecticides.

NATURALLY OCCURRING TOXICANTS

(1) Lathyrogens: Lathyrus sativus (*Khesari dhal*), is a legume (family fabaceae) commonly grown for human consumption and livestock feed in Asia and East Africa. It is a particularly important crop in areas that are prone to drought and famine, and is thought of as an 'insurance crop' as it produces reliable yields when all other crops fail. Like other grain legumes, L. sativus produces a high-protein seed. However, the seeds also contain variable amounts of a neurotoxic amino acid, β-N-Oxalyl-L-α, β-diaminopropionic acid or ODAP or BOAA. ODAP is considered as the cause of the disease neurolathyrism, a neurodegenerative disease that causes paralysis of the lower limbs: emaciation of gluteal muscle (buttocks). The disease caused by Lathyrus sativus is known as Lathyrism and the agents causing it are termed as lathyrogens.

Lathyrism:

i. Lathyrism or neurolathyrism is a neurological disease of humans and domestic animals, caused by eating certain legumes of the genus *Lathyrus*. This problem is mainly associated with *Lathyrus sativus* (also known as *Grass pea, Kesari dhal, Khesari dhal* or *Almorta*) and to a lesser degree with *Lathyrus cicera, Lathyrus ochrus* and *Lathyrus clymenum* containing the toxin ODAP. The lathyrism resulting from the ingestion of *Lathyrus odoratus* seeds (*sweet peas*) is often referred to as **odoratism** or osteolathyrism, which is caused by a different toxin (beta-aminopropionitrile) that affects the linking of collagen, a protein of connective tissues.

ii. The disease is common in Bihar, Uttar Pradesh and Madhya Pradesh as well as Spain, Algeria, France and Italy.

Symptoms:

a. In the beginning, weakness in the lower limbs with a spasticity of leg muscles. As a result, the movement of the ankle and knee joints is restricted and painful.

b. Flexion of the knee is prominent in the secondary stage and there is inversion on foot with a tendency to walk on toes.

c. In the third stage, the above symptoms become more prominent and the individual can walk only with the help of stick (Fig. 15.1).

d. In the fourth stage, the knee becomes completely flexed and walking becomes quite impossible. The thigh and leg muscles atrophy.

(2) Goitrogens:

a. The goitrogens are compounds which cause goiter. Most of them are anti-thyroid compounds or thyroid antagonists.

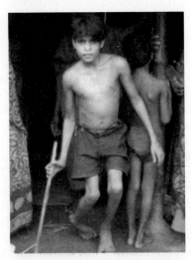

Fig. 15.1: A child suffering from lathyrism

b. Many food stuffs contain organic compounds which have goitrogenic properties.

c. The active goitrogenic principle present in the plants of brassicae family (cabbage and turnip) is 1, 5–vinyl-2-thio-oxazolidone.

d. Certain oil seeds namely, rapeseed, mustard seeds, etc. contain thioglycoside which acts as a goitrogens.

e. The red skin of groundnut contains phenolic glycosides which possess goitrogenic properties.

(3) Pressure amines:

a. A number of amines namely, histamine, tyramine, serotonin or nor-epinephrine found in some foods have profound physiological activity. Most of them are inactivated by mono-amine oxidase in the intestinal tract. The poisonous effect of pressure amines due to consumption of aged cheese has been reported in patient receiving mono-amine oxidase inhibiting drugs.

b. In Africa, the serotonin intake from plantain as a staple food may reach to 100–200 mg per day. The endomyocardial fibrosis may occur as result of large amount of serotonin.

c. The food containing pressure amines are juices of pineapples, tomatoes, bananas, lemons, etc. but mainly plaintain (green and ripe).

(4) Argemone seed oil: During the harvest of rapeseed, argemone seeds are mixed up with rapeseed which grows as weeds. The rapeseed oil obtained from a mixture of rapeseeds and argemone seeds cause epidemic dropsy (edema) in man. Apart from this, accidental or deliberate contamination of mustard oil with argemone (which is non-edible) is responsible for this toxicity. Argemone oil has carcinogenic effect when it is added at 1–2% levels to mustard oil. The toxic effects of argemone oil are due to the presence of an alkaloid, sanguinarine.

Argemone oil poisoning has been reported in the past in Delhi population after consumption of mustard oil adulterated with argemone oil, by unscrupulous traders.

A patient suffering from argemone oil poisoning is shown in Fig. 15.2.

(5) Some other toxicants of food: Some other normally occurring toxicants present in food are listed in Table 15.1.

TOXICANTS FROM PATHOGENIC MICRO-ORGANISMS

Fungal contamination: The fungi, Aspergillus flavus, Penicillium islandicum, Fusariums, Claviceps purpurae (ergot) produce a good number of toxic compounds called microtoxins.

Aspergillus flavus: This fungus has been found to be grown in cotton seeds, cereals, moist groundnuts and soya bean. It produces a toxic substance named as aflatoxin which can develop cancer and cirrhosis of the liver. The aflatoxin poisoning has recently occurred in Rajasthan and Gujarat owing to consumption of maize highly contaminated with Aspergillus flavus.

Claviceps purpurae (ergot): This parasitic fungus infects food grains such as rye and pear millet during cultivation. The disease called 'Ergotism' occurs as a result of the consumption of the contaminated

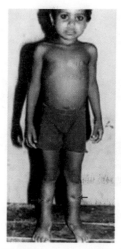

Fig.15.2: A child showing argemone oil poisoning (see edema on legs)

grains. The fungus produces the toxic alkaloids which causes the disease (ergotamines). The symptoms of this disease are nausea, vomiting, diarrhea, giddiness, severe burning sensation in extremities, painful cramps in limbs, gangrene in the fingers (Fig. 15.3) and toes, depression, weakness and convulsions.

CONTAMINATION OF FOOD WITH TOXIC CHEMICALS, PESTICIDES AND INSECTICIDES

The chemicals can contaminate food by the following ways:

Table 15.1: Some common toxicants present in food

Food	Toxicants	Biological action
Potatoes	Solanine	Interferes with transmission of nerve impulse
Lime beans, almonds	Cyanide	Inhibits cytochrome oxidase
Spinach	Oxalate	Interferes in calcium and iron absorption
Cereals	Phytate	Interferes in iron and calcium absorption
Orange peel	Citral	Binds calcium, iron and zinc to prevent their absorption
Linseed meal	Linetin	Vitamin A antagonist
TB drugs	INH	Vitamin B_6 antagonist
Sweet Cloves	Dicumarol	Vitamin K antagonist
Egg whites	Avidin	Biotin antagonist

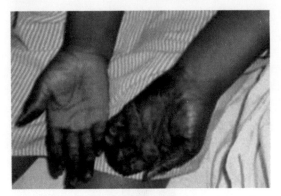

Fig. 15.3: A patient showing signs of ergotism (gangrene in the fingers)

Food additives: A large number of additives are used especially in packaged food. A food additive is defined as any substance that is not inherent part of prepared food, but is added to increase its nutritional quotient, to preserve freshness (e.g. antioxidants, antimicrobial agents), to make it taste better (e.g. sugar and salt) or look better (e.g. color). The food additives account less than 1% of the weight of humans' dietary intake. However, they play an important and beneficial role in food industry. A large variety of chemicals are added to food for many worthwhile or indispensable functions. Without food additives, it would be impossible for food to be safely produced and transported nationwide or worldwide. As preservatives, they can be categorized into three general types: antibacterial that inhibits growth of bacteria, yeasts or molds; antioxidants that show air oxidation of fats and lipids, which otherwise leads to rancidity; and a third type that blocks the enzymatic processes of natural ripening which continue to occur in food stuffs after harvest. Table 15.2 describes various uses of food additives.

1. The toxic chemicals such as barium carbonate, arsenic oxides, lead arsenate, etc. used as rat poison are accidently mixed with food.
2. Accidental contamination of food with pesticides and insecticides.
3. Some toxic chemicals or minerals are also present in certain marine foods.
4. The presence of large amount of certain food additives.

Table 15.2: Some common food additives

Categories	Examples
1. Preservative Antioxidant Antimicrobial agents	BHA (butylated hydroxyanisole) BHT Tocopherol Sodium benzoate, sodium nitrite
2. Emulsifier	Lecithin; egg yolk
3. Stabilizers and thickeners	Pectin
4. Coloring agents	Carotene; caramel
5. Flavor enhancers	Vanillin, monosodium glutamate
6. Nutrient supplements	Vitamin, iron, iodide
7. Leavening agents	Yeast, baking powder
8. Anticaking agents	Ammonium citrate, baking powder
9. Non-nutritive sweetners	Aspartame

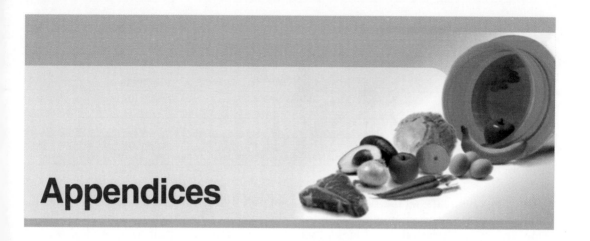

Appendices

Certain topics which have already been studied by the students are given in the appendices so that they can refresh their knowledge.

Appendix 1

INTRODUCTION TO BIOCHEMISTRY

Biochemistry like other branches of medicine comes under Science. In the simplest words, "Science is accumulated systematized knowledge especially when it relates to physical world".

There are numerous diverse things present in the world around us, so science can be sub-divided into various branches depending on the object of our study.

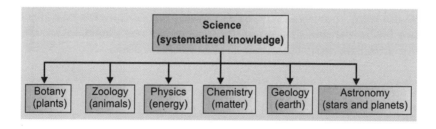

When the object of study is matter, the science is called chemistry which can be classified into various sub-branches on the basis of the nature of matter under study.

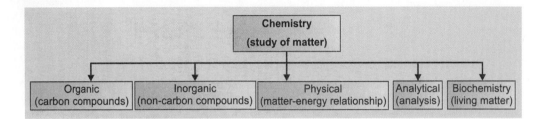

Thus, biochemistry as the name implies (bio = life) means the chemistry of living things in contrast to non-living things which are studied in other branches of chemistry.

The basic difference between living and non-living things lies in their constituent structural unit. The smallest structural unit of non-living things is a molecule, while the basic unit of the structure of the living things is a cell, which is itself composed of several molecules; so all forms of living matter are ultimately composed of cell.

Since there is variety of life forms, biochemistry, too, is of several types.

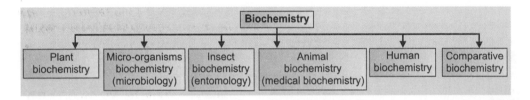

A dental student is concerned about the study of human biochemistry or medical biochemistry. This is also known as physiological chemistry. The term 'biochemistry' was introduced by Carl Neuberg in 1903.

Relationship of Biochemistry to Anatomy and Physiology

It is clear that human body is the object of study of medical biochemistry. Human body is also studied in anatomy and physiology. Then what is the difference between them? The difference lies in the angle of study. If we study the structure (gross as well as microscopic) of the human body, it is called *Anatomy*. If we study the functions (cell, tissue or organ level) of the human body, it is known as *Physiology*. *Biochemistry* is much more subtle; it goes much deeper. It probes the structure and functions of human body at the molecular level. After all, a cell is ultimately composed of molecules; a tissue is a collection of a large number of similar or dissimilar cells, and an organ is made up of numerous tissues. Smooth, orderly working of these constituent molecules is the state of health. Any derangement in the structure or function of component molecules is reflected in a disease state.

Appendix 2

CELL: STRUCTURE AND FUNCTIONS

As discussed in the previous chapter, cell is the smallest structural and functional unit of the living system. It is, therefore, appropriate to begin the study of biochemistry with the study of the cell.

Living cells may be sub-divided into two groups: Prokaryotes and Eukaryotes.

Prokaryotes: These cells lack a well defined nucleus and possess relatively simple structure, e.g. bacteria and blue-green algae.

Eukaryotes: Possess well defined nucleus and are more complex in their structure and function, e.g. animal and plant cells.

In this book, discussion will be centered only on animal cell (human cell).

The eukaryotic cells have a membrane bound nucleus and other sub-cellular organelles (Fig. A2.1), each of which has a specific function.

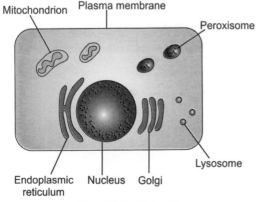

Fig. A2.1: The cell

PLASMA MEMBRANE

The plasma membrane is the outer membrane of the cell in contact with the extracellular fluid. It is responsible for maintaining constancy of the *milieu interior*. The selective permeability is an important property of plasma membrane. It is also involved in communication with other cells through binding of molecules (hormones) to receptor proteins on its surface. The plasma membrane is also involved in the secretion (exocytosis) and internalization (endocytosis) of macromolecules.

Exocytosis: Vesicles from the cytoplasm fuse with the plasma membrane, which then ruptures to release the contents (Fig. A2.2b).

Endocytosis: It involves the uptake of substances by invagination of the plasma membrane (Fig. A2.2c).

Like all biological membranes, the plasma membrane is composed of a lipid bilayer about 5 nm thick, with inserted proteins and glycoproteins (Fig. A2.3).

NUCLEUS

This is the largest organelle in the cell, being 2–10 μm in diameter. It stores the cell's genetic information as DNA in chromosomes. The nucleus is surrounded by the **nuclear envelope**, which consists of an outer membrane, which is continuous with the endoplasmic reticulum bearing attached ribosomes, and an inner membrane, separated by a gap of 15–30 nm (Fig. A2.4). The nucleus contains several thousand nuclear pores which function in the transfer

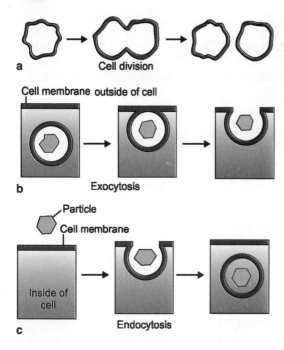

a   Cell division

b   Exocytosis

c   Endocytosis

Fig. A2.2a to c: Cell division, exocytosis and endocytosis

of molecules in and out of nucleus. A sub-region of nucleus is the **nucleolus**, which is the site of synthesis of ribosomes. Within the nucleus, the DNA is tightly coiled around histone proteins forming chromatin fibers which is associated with nuclear lamina. The nuclear lamina is the mesh of fibrous protein lying beneath the nuclear envelope. During mitosis, chromatin is condensed into discrete structures called **chromosomes** (Fig. A2.5).

ENDOPLASMIC RETICULUM

This is an inter connecting network of membranes, in the form of tubes, parallel streets and vesicles, that may extend throughout the cytoplasm. It exists in two forms: rough and smooth.

Rough endoplasmic reticulum (RER) is situated on the cytosolic side with ribosomes (Fig. A2.6) which are engaged in the synthesis of proteins destined to be secreted from the cell or to reside in the intracellular membranes.

The **smooth endoplasmic reticulum** (SER) (Fig. A2.6) has no attached ribosomes, but contains membrane bound enzymes, particularly those included in the synthesis of fatty acids and phospholipids, and in the metabolism and detoxication of drugs. It is plentiful in liver and also in muscle, where it has an important function in the accumulation of Ca^{++} after muscle contraction.

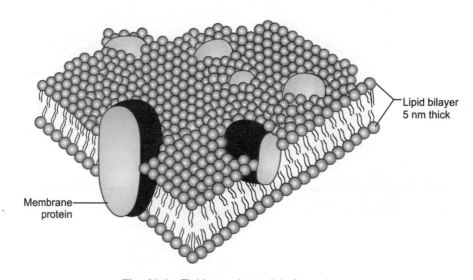

Fig. A2.3: Fluid mosaic model of membrane

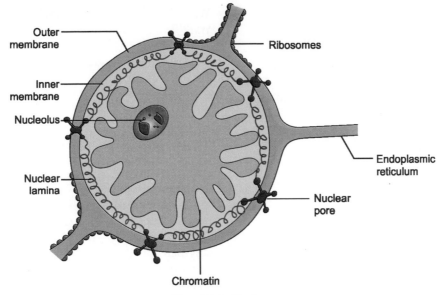

Fig. A2.4: Nucleus

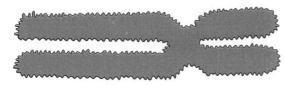

Fig. A2.5: Chromosome

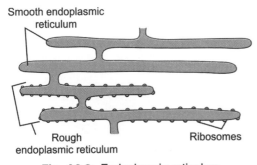

Fig. A2.6: Endoplasmic reticulum

GOLGI APPARATUS

The Golgi apparatus is a stack of flattened membrane-bound sacs. It is the sorting centre of the cell. Membrane vesicles from the RER, containing membrane and secretory proteins, fuse with the Golgi apparatus, and release their contents into it. On transit through the Golgi apparatus, further post-translational modifications (glycosylation, acylation, sulfation) of these proteins take place and they are then sorted and packaged into different vesicles. These vesicles bud off from the Golgi apparatus and are transported through the cytosol, eventually fusing either with the plasma membrane to release their contents into the extracellular space (exocytosis) or with other internal organelles (lysosomes, peroxisomes, etc.).

MITOCHONDRIA

Mitochondria have an inner and an outer membrane separated by the inter membrane space, which is about 6.5 nm (Fig. A2.7). The outer membrane is more permeable than the inner membrane due to the presence of porin proteins. The inner membrane is folded to form cristae. The inner surface of the cristae are closely packed with 8.5 nm particles, which are the sites of oxidative phosphorylation, producing ATP. Hence,

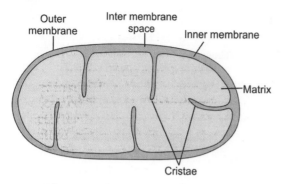

Fig. A2.7: Structure of mitochondria

the mitochondria are often called the power house of the cell. The central matrix is the site of fatty acid degradation and the citric acid cycle.

LYSOSOMES

Lysosomes have a single boundary membrane. They are a heterogeneous population of large membranous vesicles (about 1μm in diameter) formed by budding off from the Golgi apparatus. They contain hydrolytic enzymes that are maximally active at acidic pH and carry out the degradation of proteins, nucleic acids, lipids and carbohydrates. The interior of the lysosomes is maintained at pH 4.5–5.0 by ATP-driven proton translocation from the cytoplasm. Lysosomes are responsible for the degradation of macromolecules taken into the cells by endocytosis, and for the complete destruction of cellular structure after cell death.

PEROXISOMES

These are small (0.2–1.0 μm) membrane-bounded organelles, which have a single boundary membrane and contain enzymes that degrade fatty acids and amino acids. A by-product of these reactions is hydrogen peroxide which is toxic to the cell. The presence of large amounts of the enzyme catalase in the peroxisomes rapidly converts the toxic H_2O_2 into harmless water and oxygen.

CYTOPLASM

The intracellular space surrounding the cell organelles is the cytoplasm. Strictly speaking, this consists of all the components of a cell apart from the nucleus.

CYTOSOL

This is the part of the cell which is devoid of organized components (organelles). It contains a large number of different enzymes and proteins, and is a major site of cellular metabolism. The cytosol is not homogeneous but has within it the cytoskeleton, a network of fibers criss-crossing through the cell that helps to maintain its shape (Fig. A2.8). The cytoskeleton lattice includes three types of fibers: microtubules (diameter, 25 nm) based on the protein tubulin, intermediate filaments (diameter, 10 nm) and microfilament (diameter, 8 nm) based on the protein actin. Apart from these, also found within the cytosol of many cells are inclusion bodies (granules of material that are not membrane-bound) such as glycogen granules in liver and muscle cells,

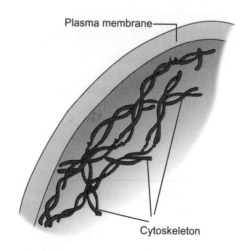

Fig. A2.8: Cytoskeleton of red cells

and droplets of fat in the cells of adipose tissue.

All the three types of fibers are formed by the polymerization of relatively small protein monomers. Microtubules are involved in the maintenance of the cell shape, in the movement of chromosomes and other sub-cellular components, and in propelling of motile cells (such as spermatozoa). Microfilaments are involved in cell division, endocytosis, exocytosis (Fig. A2.2), cell locomotion, the maintenance of cell shape (an example of which is brush border of the intestinal cells). The function of intermediate filaments is not fully understood, but it may probably to confer mechanical strength and stability. Thus, keratin filaments are plentiful in epithelial cells. Examples are the skin and the lining of the intestine.

METABOLIC FUNCTIONS OF ORGANELLES

The various compartments of the cell have different assigned functions. This is listed in Table A2.1.

Table A2.1: Cell organelles and their functions

Organelles	Functions
Plasma membrane	Cell recognition, cell signalling, transport mechanisms
Nucleus	Nucleic acid synthesis
Rough endoplasmic reticulum	Protein synthesis
Smooth endoplasmic reticulum	Lipid metabolism, drug metabolism
Golgi apparatus	Packaging of secretory proteins and lysosomal enzymes
Mitochondria	Oxidation of fatty acids, TCA cycle, part of urea cycle, electron transport and oxidative phosphorylation, control of cytosolic Ca^{++} levels, ketone body synthesis
Lysosomes	Proteolytic enzymes
Peroxisomes	Oxidation leading to H_2O_2 production and its decomposition by catalase
Cytosol	Glycolysis, HMP shunt, gluconeogenesis

Appendix 3

ACID–BASE BALANCE

The cell and body fluids contain numerous substances which may be acidic, basic or neutral. Their relative quantity determines the final pH. One of the prerequisites of normal functioning of cells is the maintenance of almost neutral pH of their interior. This is achieved by a few buffers. Buffer solutions are generally made of weak acids and their salts of strong base. Such solutions have the ability to accept H^+ and OH^- ions without undergoing any pH change.

Buffers have an important role to play in restricting pH changes of body fluids. Buffers act as shock absorbers against sudden changes of pH by converting injurious strong acids and bases into harmless weak acid salts.

Physiological Buffers

Some of the major buffering systems of body are described below:

Buffers of the plasma: Plasma has three buffer systems.

i. Carbonic acid-bicarbonate (H_2CO_3/ $BHCO_3$): It is the most important buffering system of the plasma and is present in fairly high concentration ($H_2CO_3 = 0.0025M$ and $BHCO_3 = 0.025M$). The ratio of $H_2CO_3/BHCO_3$ in plasma is 1/20 which gives a pH of 7.4.

ii. Plasma protein buffer system (B-Protein/ H-Protein): Plasma proteins being amphoteric compounds act both as acceptors and donors of H^+ ions and thus play an important role in regulating the pH of the blood.

iii. Phosphate buffer system (B_2HPO_4/ BH_2PO_4): It is a weak and less important buffer system of blood plasma. The ratio of B_2HPO_4/BH_2PO_4 is 4:1.

Buffers of red blood cells: In erythrocytes also, different buffering systems function. These are described below.

i. Carbonic acid-bicarbonate (H_2CO_3/ $BHCO_3$): As in plasma, this system has quantitative importance in erythrocytes.

ii. Oxyhemoglobinate-oxyhemoglobin system ($BHbO_2/HHbO_2$) and

iii. Hemoglobinate-hemoglobin system (BHb/HHb): In both buffering systems, oxyhemoglobin and hemoglobin play the role of maintaining pH by acting as amphoteric substances.

Buffers of tissue fluids and tissues: The buffering system of lymph, spinal fluid, etc. are similar to that of blood though much less in quantity.

The buffering capacity in tissues is due to $H_2CO_3/BHCO_3$ system, protein buffers and organic acid/salt systems, out of this $H_2CO_3/BHCO_3$ is the chief buffering system in these fluids.

Parameters Affecting pH of Blood

The pH of blood depends upon a large number of acidic and basic substances, the most important of which are two—carbonic acid and the bicarbonate. Carbonic acid is formed by the hydration of carbon dioxide, which is liberated by the cellular metabolism and the bicarbonate is produced by dissociation of carbonic acid.

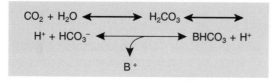

$$CO_2 + H_2O \rightleftharpoons H_2CO_3 \rightleftharpoons$$

$$H^+ + HCO_3^- \rightleftharpoons BHCO_3 + H^+$$

$$B^+$$

where B^+ represents cations in the blood, principally Na^+ and K^+.

The relative proportions of carbonic acid to bicarbonate (1:20) determines the pH of the blood, which is 7.40 in case of venous blood as against 7.43 of the arterial blood.

As long as the ratio of carbonic acid to bicarbonate in the blood is 1:20, the pH of the blood remains normal. Any alteration in this ratio will disturb the acid–base balance of the blood and tissues towards acidosis or alkalosis. Obviously, the ratio can be altered either by the alteration in H_2CO_3 content or bicarbonate ($BHCO_3$) content.

Alterations in the H_2CO_3 Content

The content of H_2CO_3 in the blood is under the control of the respiratory system because of the dependence of carbonic acid on the partial pressure of CO_2 (pCO_2), which in turn is controlled by the organs of respiratory system (lungs). As a result, disturbances in acid–base balance which are due to alterations in the content of H_2CO_3 of the blood are said to be respiratory in origin. Thus, respiratory acidosis will occur when there is an accumulation of H_2CO_3 in the blood; conversely respiratory alkalosis will occur when the rate of elimination of CO_2 is excessive, so that a reduction of H_2CO_3 occurs in the blood. In either case, the normal 1:20 ratio of H_2CO_3 to $BHCO_3$ is disturbed and the pH of the blood will fall or rise in accordance with the retention or the excessive elimination of CO_2.

Role of the Kidneys in Acid–Base Balance

If the bicarbonate content of the blood can be adjusted to restore the 1:20 ratio between carbonic acid and bicarbonate, the pH will once more return to normal. Such an adjustment is accomplished by the kidneys in respiratory acidosis by reabsorption of more bicarbonate in the renal tubules and in respiratory alkalosis by excreting more bicarbonate in the urine. The respiratory acidosis or alkalosis is then said to be compensated, which means that even though the amounts of H_2CO_3 and $BHCO_3$ in the blood are abnormal, the pH is normal because the ratio of the two has been restored to the normal 1:20. The CO_2 content of the plasma (pCO_2) will be higher than normal in compensated respiratory acidosis and lower than normal in compensated respiratory alkalosis.

Alterations in the Bicarbonate Content

Disturbances in acid–base balance which are due to alterations in the content of bicarbonate in the blood are said to be metabolic in origin. A deficit of bicarbonate without any change in H_2CO_3 will be metabolic acidosis and excess of bicarbonate, a metabolic alkalosis.

Role of Lungs in Acid–Base Balance

Correction of pH will occur by adjustment of H_2CO_3 concentration, in the former case by elimination of more CO_2 (hyperventilation) and in the latter case by retention of CO_2 (depressed respiration). The CO_2 content of the plasma (pCO_2) will obviously be lower than normal in metabolic acidosis and higher than normal in metabolic alkalosis.

CAUSES OF DISTURBANCE IN ACID–BASE BALANCE

There are various causes of disturbances in acid-base balance of the body. These are described below.

(a) Metabolic Acidosis

It is caused by a decrease in the bicarbonate fraction, with either no change or relatively smaller change in the carbonic acid fraction.

This is most common type of acidosis. It occurs in:

i. Uncontrolled diabetes mellitus, due to accumulation of acidic ketone bodies
ii. Cases of vomiting when fluids lost are not acidic
iii. Renal disease
iv. Poisoning by acidic salt
v. Excessive losses of intestinal fluids (diarrhea or colitis)
vi. Excessive losses of electrolytes.

Increased respiration (hyperpnea) is an important sign of an uncompensated acidosis.

(b) Respiratory Acidosis

It is caused by an increase in carbonic acid relative to bicarbonate. It may occur in any disease which impairs respiration, such as:

i. Pneumonia
ii. Emphysema
iii. Congestive heart failure
iv. Asthma
v. Depression of respiratory centre (as by morphine poisoning).

(c) Metabolic Alkalosis

It occurs when there is an increase in the bicarbonate fraction, with either no change or relatively smaller change in the carbonic acid fraction. This may occur in:

i. Ingestion of large quantities of alkali such as in patients of peptic ulcer on antacid therapy
ii. Intestinal obstruction as in pyloric stenosis
iii. Prolonged vomiting
iv. Cushing's disease.

The raised blood pH of an uncompensated alkalosis often leads to tetany, possibly owing to decrease in ionized serum calcium.

In all types of uncompensated alkalosis, the respirations are slow and shallow and the urine may be alkaline.

(d) Respiratory Alkalosis

It occurs when there is a decrease in the carbonic acid fraction with no corresponding change in bicarbonate. This occurs in:

i. Hysterical hyperventilation
ii. CNS diseases affecting respiratory system
iii. Early stages of salicylate poisoning
iv. Hyperpnea observed at high altitude.

Appendix 4

IMMUNOGLOBULINS

The immunoglobulins are antibodies which are present in plasma as a part of gamma globulins.

ANTIBODIES

Antibodies are constituents of body fluids either normally present or produced by introduction of an antigenic substance in the body. Chemically antibodies are glycoproteins and are called immunoglobulins.

ANTIGEN

An antigen is a substance which after introduction into human or animal body is capable of producing defensive substances (antibodies) and inducing immunity. Almost any class of organic compound may be antigenic, especially macromolecules of proteins and carbohydrates.

IMMUNOGLOBULINS

The immunoglobulins constitute a heterogenous family of serum proteins which either functions as antibodies or are chemically related to them. Immunoglobulins are divided into five main classes on the basis of their structures—IgG, IgA, IgM, IgD and IgE. There are further subclasses of each of these immunoglobulins.

IMMUNOGLOBULIN STRUCTURE

The immunoglobulins are Y-shaped, symmetrical protein molecules composed of pairs of two identical polypeptide chains, joined together by a disulphide bond. The two identical chains are called light (L) and heavy (H) chains. Light chain has about 220 amino acids and heavy chain about 440 amino acids. Each light chain has a variable region at N-terminal end which is different in different immunoglobulins and constant region at its C-terminal which is made of same amino acids. Similarly, each heavy chain has an N-terminal variable region and C-terminal constant region. The N-terminal ends of one heavy chain and its neighboring light chain cooperate to form an antigen-binding site, so that IgG molecule has two binding sites for antigen. Thus, it can bind two molecules of antigen, hence, it is bivalent (the valency is two). Disulphide bonds join together the two heavy chains as well as constant region of each heavy chain with its neighboring light chain. Apart from these interchain disulphide bonds, there is intrachain disulphide bonds in both the light as well as the heavy chains. The immunoglobulin molecule has carbohydrate which is linked to the heavy chain (Fig. A4.1).

Since it is the variable region of both the light and heavy chains which make up antigen-binding site, the variability in amino acid sequence of these regions explains how different sites with different specificities for antigen binding can be formed. In the three dimensional structure of the immunoglobulin molecule, the variable parts of the light and heavy chains are looped together to form the antigen binding site. A single antibody molecule combines with two antigen molecules and so cross-link and precipitate antigen out.

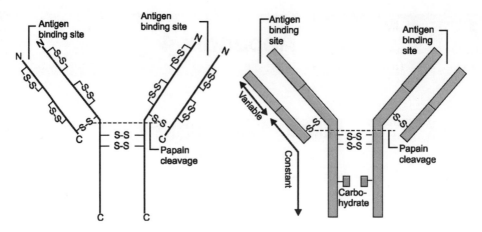

Fig. A4.1: Immunoglobulin structure showing (left) disulphide bonds (right) variable and constant regions

The variable regions of opposed heavy and light chains create a pocket of unique three-dimensional internal forms, into which a part of antigen molecule can fit closely and bind tightly.

CLASSIFICATION OF IMMUNOGLOBULINS

Although two different forms of light chains exist—'kappa' (k) or 'lambda' (λ) but in an antibody molecule, either two k light chains (M.wt = 23,000) or two λ light chains (M.wt = 23,000) can be present. On the other hand, five different heavy chains have been identified in immunoglobulins. Hence, their classification is based on the form of H-chain present. Their molecular weight varies from 50,000 to 70,000. Humans have five different classes of immunoglobulin molecules which differ both in structure and function.

These are:

Immunoglobulin	H-chain
IgA	alpha (α)
IgD	delta (δ)
IgE	epsilon (ε)
IgG	gamma (γ)
IgM	mu (μ)

Carbohydrate Content of Immunoglobulins

All immunoglobulins are glycoproteins and their carbohydrate content varies substantially. The carbohydrate moieties are heteropolysaccharides which are primarily linked to asparagine. Table A4.1 shows the carbohydrate content of some of the immunoglobulins.

Table A4.1: Carbohydrate content of immunoglobulins						
Class	Galactose	Mannose	N-acetyl glucosa-mine	Sialic acid	Fucrose carbo-hydrate	Total
IgA	1.2	1.7	1.6	0.9	0.2	6.4
IgG	0.4	0.6	1.3	0.2	0.3	2.8
IgM	1.6	3.3	3.3	1.3	0.7	10.2

INDIVIDUAL IMMUNOGLOBULINS

The different heavy chains confer different properties and functions on each of the immunoglobulin classes.

IgM: IgM has mu (μ) heavy chains and exists as a pentamer in combination with another polypeptide, called the J-chain, which is responsible for initiating the polymerization to form the pentameric structure. With its large number of antigen binding sites, each IgM molecule binds very tightly to any pathogen. The binding also activates the complement pathway and macrophages. Therefore, IgM is the first antibody produced when an animal responds to a new antigen.

IgG: IgG is the main immunoglobulin in the blood in late primary immune response and during secondary immune response. Like IgM, it can activate complement and trigger macrophages. It is the only antibody that can pass through the placenta and so provide immunological protection for the fetus. It is also secreted into the mother's milk and is absorbed by the gut of the newborn, thus providing continued protection after birth.

IgA: IgA is the main class of immunoglobulin in secretion such as tears, saliva and in secretion of the lungs and the intestine. It is the first line of immunological defense against infection at these sites.

IgE: IgE occurs in tissues where, after binding the antigen, it stimulates mast cells to release and activate eosinophils to kill various types of parasites. However, the mast cells can also release histamine which causes dilation and increase permeability of blood vessels and lead to symptoms seen in allergic reactions, such as hay fever and asthma.

IgD: IgD is formed on the surface of mature B-lymphocytes and in traces in various body fluids, but its exact function is not clear.

Index

Reader's Notes